MW01629940

{ IN **PURSUIT** OF }
Optimum Health

Enjoy optimum health in life—through knowledge

Your health is your choice

Phil's enthusiastic students and friends have awaited his book:

In 2012 I was diagnosed with breast cancer. My doctor recommended surgery. Phil became my life coach, giving me hope and courage in my cancer battle. The new healthy lifestyle (alternative cancer treatment) made me feel better than I had in years! Within 3 months, the lump dissipated. Six years later I'm still cancer-free and living a healthy happy life!

Thank you Phil and Evelyn, I owe you my life!

—Tammy Paul

I was diagnosed with hepatitis a few years ago and consulted with Phil who made helpful recommendations. Fasting and using Schulze herbs to detoxify my body, in about 3 months I was clear of hepatitis. I really appreciate Mr. Fons and his wisdom.

—Donni Lee Pettit, Arroyo Grande, CA

{ IN } PURSUIT OF } Optimum Health

INFORMATION COMPILED BY

PHILIP C. FONS & EVELYN FONS

In Pursuit of Optimum Health
Copyright © 2019 by Evelyn Fons

Fons, Evelyn
In Pursuit of Optimum Health: How to prevent cancer or help you heal if you already live with it.

All rights reserved. No part of this publication may be reproduced, stored in a retrieval system, or transmitted in any form or by any means—electronic, mechanical, photocopy, recording, or any other—except for brief quotations in printed reviews, without the permission of the author or the author's representative.

Published by My Write Art Place / Caroll L. (Shreeve) Riley
Printed by West Wind Litho / West Valley City, Utah
Printed in the United States of America

ISBN-13: 978-0-578-44490-1
ISBN-10: 0-578-44490-9

1. Self-Help/Health 2. Holistic Nutrition 3. Healthy Lifestyle
4. Inspiration: Cancer 5. Cookbook

Editorial Coordinator: Caroll L. (Shreeve) Riley
Cover and interior page design: Maralee Nelson / mGraphicDesign

18 19 20 21 /CLS/ 28 27 26 25 24

Fran
   appreciate all your hard work.
many people benefit from it.
     Phil & Evelyn sold the Pioneer
building to my Father and I.
     At the time I was not aware
of his prior life. Amazing.
     This book is also amazing because
I know it is true.
     The best Doctor you will ever have
is your own immune system.
                    Sincerly
                    Ed Nelson

SPECIAL NOTE

The information contained in this publication is a compilation of all the sources of information and authority researched and compiled by Phillip Fons and used for instructional purposes in his three Dixie State University classes for eight years. Some of the research references exist without the author's identity due to Phillip's unfortunate passing prior to completion of this manuscript. Evelyn has made every attempt to accurately represent all information and sources whenever possible.

TABLE *of* CONTENTS

by Pat Sapio

YEARS AGO, I suggested to Phil Fons that since he was a man of such personal conviction about people taking charge of their own health, the Institute of Continued Learning participants at Dixie State in St. George, Utah would benefit from his expertise. He followed up and taught a well-attended and enthusiastic-response class for eight years. This book has grown out of his research and lecture notes from those years.

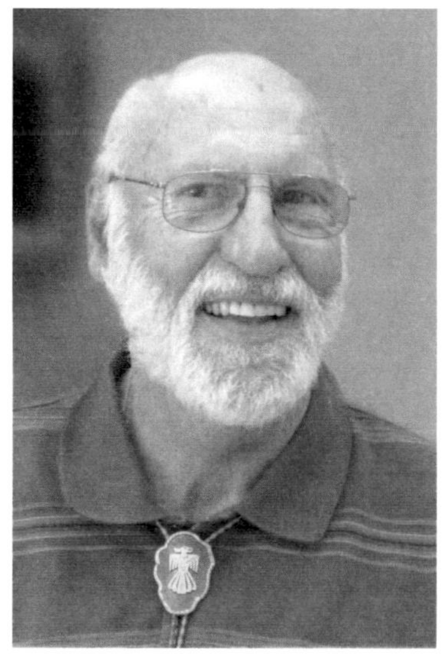

Phil was working on his manuscript with his wife, Evelyn's able assistance. Unfortunately, at age 92, he died and left her to carry on his dream of sharing his research and personal-experience results with the students who had begged him to write a book. His desire to inspire them with positive guidance for living to their highest potential physically, emotionally and spiritually fell to Evelyn to complete in book form.

In Pursuit of Optimum Health contains a wealth of practical, plain common-sense suggestions delivered in Phil's scientific yet folksy style. As a space engineer with Rocketdyne, research was his natural bent. When Evelyn was diagnosed with cancer, he consulted every study and avenue medically and holistically to cure her—without resorting to surgery, radiation and chemotherapy—if those "treatments" could be avoided.

His research, interviews and common sense led him to alternatives that called for herbal and unprocessed health-food nutrients and oxygenating the body with appropriate exercise. He also sent Evelyn to a health spa for three weeks to learn those techniques. She has been cancer-free for over thirty years! She never had surgery or endured radiation or chemotherapy. She healed herself through the techniques she learned and lives by them to this day.

Phil's popular class: "You Don't Have to Die From Cancer" expounded on his passion for being positive, treating your body with respect and support, and committing to a healthy lifestyle.

Evelyn, now at age 92 herself, is living proof that a change of lifestyle works. This book has life-saving information, much of it recorded no where else unless you personally consult the studies Phil researched.

In Pursuit of Optimum Health is crammed with suggestions for preventing life-threatening diseases and improving your quality of life for those coping with serious ailments, such as cancer.

I am honored to have been asked by Evelyn to write this foreword in support of my late colleague and friend, Phil Fons.

—Pat Sapio

MY DEAR HUSBAND, Phillip Corrigan Fons, passed away June 10, 2014, at the age of 92. He had been in a coma for several days without any response, lying on a hospital bed in front of the fireplace in our living room. A friend, who is a nurse, phoned me from Minnesota and told me to keep talking to Phil because the spirit is still there and hears. It seemed reasonable to me because the spirit is in the mortal body. I had sat talking to him, explaining how much he was loved and how the Lord needed him. Phil would have much work to do on the other side, and I promised to finish things here and I would join him as soon as possible.

My hand resting beneath his, like it had been for nearly fifty-one years, I whispered, "Honey, if you hear me, would you squeeze my hand?"

In response, the tips of his four fingers gently pressed down into my palm. My heart leaped—he'd heard me! What a tender mercy. That was our last communication.

He hadn't eaten or responded to me in several days. That next morning, around six, I awoke with an urgency to check on my husband. When he passed, I felt sad yet relieved because he was at peace, no longer bed-ridden and in a coma.

In all our extraordinary years together, my amazement for his strength and wisdom never ceased. Truly, he was a man of God and a real live rocket scientist! I am grateful to have known him and to have been his wife. I look forward to spending eternity with him.

But first, I must fulfill my promise to him to write this book for him. He wanted more than anything to make an indelible mark upon the pages of history and within the hearts and minds of those who knew and loved him. A faithful servant and natural-born teacher, he wanted to help others gain truth, goodness, and receptivity in a variety of ideas, insights, and values.

For several years, Phil taught at Dixie State College, which us now Dixie State University, for the Institute of Continual Learning (ICL). Phil had earned a teaching certificate from UCLA. I have written this book from his numerous class notes he used in teaching his classes. He was 91 when he taught his last class. One of these classes was titled "With Prevention, You Don't Have to Die from Cancer." In Chapter Two, I will share his class notes and our family experiences with fighting cancer for myself and our son.

It was Phil's goal and mine to help others find the knowledge, as we have been able to do, to have a healthier lifestyle. Our purpose in writing this book is to awaken people to the fact that we are what we eat, and he taught the things that contribute to optimum health.

I start this book the way Phil always started his classes, with the following anonymous quote:

GOOD HEALTH IS

having no fatigue

having a good appetite

going to sleep and awakening easily,

having a good memory,

having good humor,

having precision in thought and action,

being honest, humble, grateful, and loving.

The doctor of the future will have no medicine but will interest his patients in the care of the human frame, in diet, and in the cause and prevention of disease.

—Thomas A. Edison

In the chapters that follow, journey with me as I follow the prevention-and-healing guidance my husband Phil shared year after year with his students. They came to learn at his feet, and I hope you will learn from his wise advice how to lead a healthy, happy, life full of love and fulfillment.

—Evelyn Fons
Mrs. Phil Fons

INTRODUCTION:
OUR FRUITFUL PAST

*How our parents prepared us to value
achieving and maintaining optimum health.*

I REMEMBER READING that everything operates in perfect harmony for the benefit and enjoyment of all. I, also, am in awe at how the good Lord created this universe for that purpose. He created this earth, the trees and foliage, vegetables, berries, nuts, seeds and wild game—producing food for every living creature to be harvested and reproduced. He also created man and all creatures that must have sunshine, water and proper nourishment to stay healthy and to reproduce. I think of the beautiful flowers and what they mean to the little hummingbirds and bees, as it's their job to pollinate them for procreation. Every living thing reproduces after its own kind—fish and animals for meat for other species, vegetables of every sort, loaded with vitamins and minerals for man and beasts.

I remember how my pet horse loved to eat apples and carrots, how the rabbits raided our garden and how we and many other species depend upon the variety of berries, grains, vegetables and fruit that grow. I only wish we could be more grateful for all that He has provided for us and focus on all the good things in life that we enjoy. God gave us a brain and everything we need. If we could only use our minds to their full potential and advantage. There are so many challenges in life including poor or less-than-ideal health. If we could only open our minds and understand how our bodies work, and how we should take care of ourselves, then we would lead healthy, happy and productive lives.

We really are what we eat. Man has suffered multiple diseases and maladies and through research and experience learned to overcome them. This is the primary purpose in writing this book for Phil—to help others secure the knowledge we have found to help all of us help ourselves.

My husband, Phillip Corrigan Fons, was born 21 March 1922 in Chicago, Cook County, Illinois. He grew up there in Chicago where his wise mother and father always had a garden and made sure their sons had proper fresh food. We were both raised to appreciate the foods our Lord provided us, and we were happier and healthier for it.

I grew up on a ranch in Idaho where we had

good wholesome food. My father and mother really knew how to live off the land. They had a working farm that provided meats without hormones, fresh fruit in abundance and nutrient-rich vegetables, wild honey for sweetening, and fresh raw cow's milk without additives (which I only drank when my mother made me because I didn't like its flavor). My father was a farmer as well as a rancher, and I remember how he would rotate his crops. With the high demand of the population now, the same soil is used repeatedly and "enriched" with questionable chemical fertilizers. Many of them are used to force growth. I question if plants of today are as healthy or nourishing as they once were. Like the plants that need proper nourishment, so our bodies must also have proper nutrition. If the produce we eat does not contain the nutrients we need, we cannot build strong bones and bodies. With so many people suffering from illnesses now, one can't help but question the reasons why.

Dad was a proud Englishman. He took pride in raising our meat and butchering it. The meat was free of all chemicals and it was derived from animals that were fed good things. Mother too made sure we had the best healthy food. She worked hard growing a garden. We little ones helped as much as possible and learned by example. No pesticides or chemicals on our vegetables! For plants to grow, they must have fertile soil. The soil must be fertilized and mulched and requires sunshine, water and loving care.

Dad would use the fertilizer from the animal waste and also put the leftover hay and clippings in the compost over the garden and his fields in the fall, which would decompose under the snow all winter. Dad would make a pit in the ground, line it with straw and put heads of cabbage, carrots and other root crops in and cover them with straw. It would snow and cover them all winter. Whenever something would be needed for a meal, Mother would say, "Would you go out and get a cabbage or a few carrots?" I always thought "a few" meant six because we had six in our family. So one of us would go out and move the covering, covered with snow, and dig down through the straw and find what we were looking for and then recover the vegetables for protection from the freezing cold.

By spring, when it warmed up, he would plow the soil and prepare it for planting. With all the good water he would pipe from the nearby stream, we had the best garden in the country. From this, she preserved everything for winter by drying, bottling, making sauerkraut in crocks, etc. She baked our bread from a sourdough starter and made the best cookies, pies, and cakes, which we didn't have very often, and such a treat when we did. So, our intake of sugar was limited. Christmas time, of course, we always got a stocking full of the most delicious candies, nuts, and oranges. The cellar was full of potatoes, onions, apples, bottled fruit, jellies, jams, and veggies. We, of course, had our own milk, butter, cheese, and eggs from our cage-free chickens. I matured with strong bones as I ate plenty of good vegetables from the garden as well as sunflower seeds, and other natural sources of calcium.

I have a friend who drinks milk daily and yet is terribly crippled with osteoporosis. I am sure the raw, unpasteurized milk we had as children was better for us than the homogenized version full of hormones in the markets today. My mother made cheese and butter and used our milk in healthy recipes for puddings, cakes, and a variety of other foods. The entire family enjoyed the benefits of fresh milk, and even our kittens loved it!

We were fortunate during the Depression years to have all that healthy bounty when so many were in need. We didn't realize or appreciate any of it until we got older, but at least we always have had a strong understanding of what foods were best for us. Many Americans don't have the same opportunities.

CHAPTER TWO

CANCER FIRST-HAND

W HEN I WAS GROWING UP, cancer was rarely heard of, and I didn't see a doctor until I was in high school. Mother had knowledge passed down through generations on how to treat childhood ailments, and apparently it worked. We all made it. My point throughout this book is that we must be doing something wrong to have all the problems of health that we have now. Common sense tells us something is wrong, and it is up to us individually to each take our health into our own hands and be responsible for it.

We seem to feel we can take our bodies to our doctors and say "fix me" just like when we take our car to the garage and have it repaired. Don't get me wrong. I love my doctors and wouldn't want to be without them, but bless their hearts, they can't think *for* us. They can advise us and put Band-Aids on, but they can't get to the basic cause of what we are doing to ourselves, and many won't even follow their advice.

I remember a friend when we lived in California telling me she was so ill and kept going to doctors, but they couldn't help her. She wasn't improving. She had a family to care for and needed to be well for them. She was praying one evening, and a voice said to her, "Eat all of your food raw." She never knew this was possible! But she was desperate to get well. She did this, and her body healed itself. I had always remembered her experience.

When I was told, after being ill for quite a long time and the doctor couldn't find my problem until I had a biopsy, which showed cancer cells, I recalled my friend's cure. With my husband, I began to study all we could find out about the benefits of consuming raw foods. The following are some things we learned:

Raw foods in a diet provide needed enzymes and act as a broom helping to cleanse and sweep the intestinal tract, removing waste matter from the colon. Cooked and processed foods are dead foods that promote the accumulation of toxic matter in the colon.

I think by now, we know that the American medical system isn't necessarily set up to nurse you back to health. It's more for diagnosing and managing the symptoms of diseases, not preventing or curing them.

We even learned from Johnathon Landsman, host of an Oral Health online event that root-canal procedures increase your risk of cancer and other degenerative diseases. He says we can begin to reverse some types of cancer by reducing oral infections.

Back decades ago, everyone died of cancer. I was prepared to die too. However, my dear husband, the rocket scientist that he was, listened to a friend who came over to visit us. Upon hearing the news of my diagnosis, he told us that while fighting colon cancer he had gone to a place in San Diego, called Optimum Health Institute and had been able to overcome his cancer.

My husband was on the phone immediately making reservations for me to go. I reluctantly went, thinking, "I want to be home when I die." My dear friend Mikiko went with me. It was a beautiful place, so serene and pristine. A peaceful feeling engulfed me, and I loved it.

Not knowing what I was in for, I was pleasantly surprised to learn that it was not their responsibility to heal me. It was up to me. I would be taught correct principals, and it was up to me to heal myself! They informed us that they can't cure anything. All they do is teach us better alternatives to our lifestyles.

The cleansing program, referred to as Phase I, is a three-week detoxification program for the body. Depending upon the health challenges it may be necessary to remain on Phase I for three to six months. Their Optimal Living Recipes are the mainstays of cleansing and life renewing. When the body is cleansed to the degree that the person feels energetic, vital, joyful, and enthusiastic, then (and only then) may introduce other cooked foods. They are considered transitional foods, which are to be eaten in moderation.

Also, because cancer doesn't thrive in oxygen; we were encouraged to perform an arm-lifting exercise of inhaling deeply while raising our arms above our heads. Exhale as you lower your arms. Repeat 10 reps each time, several times a day for maximum oxygenating benefit at the cell level. The whole idea is to help our bodies heal themselves.

I couldn't help but wonder as I went through some of the lectures and classes, why isn't this taught in our schools? It should be mandatory. They do have health classes all compiled by statistics from the government manufacturing profiling. So much money is spent on saving the hoot owl and other species, so why can't they put dollars aside for educating us on how to keep our bodies healthy?

The first week in my program at Optimum Health Institute was detoxing, helping my body to detox and get more alkaline so it could fight back against my cancer. We learned that when the body is in the acidic mode, it is subject to illnesses. After the first week, I did feel so much better, and I began to feel like I would actually live.

I learned so much about how the body works and what happens in the body if not properly nourished with food and exercise. I spent three weeks in this wonderful place.

My dear husband came and joined me for the third week and was amazed at how I had progressed. I will always be grateful to the friend who told us about this healing option that had worked for him and for this opportunity being available to help me get well.

The gray color of my skin disappeared. I stayed on the regime that I had learned for over a year and then as they suggested, I began to gradually add cooked foods back into my meals. If you prefer to do so, be sure that you eat 80 percent raw and 20 percent cooked food. I try to follow this even now and my cancer has never returned. I have gone back many times over 30 years—for two weeks each time—to detox, relearn and to have a nice restorative vacation in beautiful surroundings.

My husband, learning with me and seeing what happened and being the researcher that he was, began his quest of learning about cancer. He did much of his research at the CHIC center at our Dixie Medical Hospital here in our little town of St. George, Utah, which was well known for the expertise that it offered and the wonderful doctors on staff. He was asked by our friend Pat Sapio connected with Dixie State College, now Dixie State University, to teach a class for the Institute of Continued Learning (ICL) on his findings, and this he did along with what he had learned about heart problems that I inherited, present at birth, and tried to overcome.

There are so many things we can do to have healthy families. We learned so much during our battle with cancer, and I do mean battle as I wanted to live and my husband did constant research.

Phil and I both talked with Bill Henderson on several occasions when our son was suffering with prostate cancer. Bill was a great man and helped so many. Little did Bill know that the next month he would be diagnosed with non-Hodgkin's lymphoma (NHL), which is a form of cancer that starts in the lymphocytes. Over the past half year, Bill had been successfully utilizing multiple natural treatment protocols, with visible results and lab report improvement, steadily gaining momentum against the malignancy. However, Bill's form of NHL required frequent blood transfusions, especially platelets. The problem was that he also had thrombophlebitis, which resulted in blood clots in his legs. According to the physician who was treating Bill, it was a combination of heart attack, stroke, and pulmonary embolism in the wake of a blood transfusion, which took his life. We learned about his passing on the Internet and it made us very sad. It was *not* due to cancer.

Bill's widow, Terry, stepped into his shoes to honor his legacy and continue his work. Bill's most popular book is *Cancer-Free—Your Guide to Gentle, Non-Toxic Healing*.

I know how frightening it is to be told you have cancer, but read what has been written about what you need to know concerning the dangers of chemotherapy and radiation and why cancer is big business. We are not in control of what the media tells us about cancer treatment, and the causes of cancer and how we can reverse these conditions and get well if we so choose to learn and be knowledgeable and find there is hope.

It is critical that you clearly understand your diagnosis and the proposed treatment. Ask your doctor these following questions and note the answers for later reference:

· Precisely what type of cancer do I have?

· Has the cancer spread beyond the primary site? Where?

· What tests did you use to determine this
diagnosis?

· Is there any indication that a second
pathology report is needed?

· Do you recommend additional tests?
Looking for what?

· Are you certain tests & resulting diagnoses are
accurate?

· What are my treatment options? Which
one(s) do you recommend?
(Record these recommendations in precise detail)

· Will you obtain and review with me the
treatment information on my type and stage
of cancer from the National Cancer Institute's
Physicians Data Query (PDQ) program?

· Whom do you recommend for a second
opinion?

· Are you a board-certified oncologist?

CHAPTER THREE

WITH PREVENTION, YOU DON'T HAVE TO DIE FROM CANCER

IN MY INTRODUCTION, you may recall that Phil taught a class titled "With Prevention, You Don't Have to Die from Cancer." As a cancer survivor of for over 30 years myself—without radiation, chemo or surgery—I benefited from his research and support. I know the information provided in that class is of critical importance in the prevention and battle to achieve cancer remission. Cancer is a scourge on our society and many readers of this book will be grateful for Phil's research in their own prevention and battle plans to combat cancer.

Phil researched and found cancer to be the second leading cause of death in America today. Yet, people from all over the world are successfully using alternative means to prevent and overcome cancer. The three conventional treatments for cancer are chemotherapy, radiation and surgery, which have been used for the past fifty years—yet nothing has prevented cancer, and it is even more prevalent today. Attempts are made to overcome or delay it but America seems to be losing the war on cancer. Nearly every day, when I read the obituaries, someone has died after battling cancer. Now, even our children are dying from it.

Dr. Schulze, natural healing advocate, indicates "...cancer is caused by environmental toxins and poisons. It has been said that 80 percent of all cancers are a direct result of chemicals in our air, water and food based on information according to leading experts. Of those 70,000 chemicals, less than 7 percent have been tested for adverse effects." These environmental toxins are present everywhere from our food to our water, to the air we breathe. Even cosmetics, in contact with our skin, allow the chemicals to go directly into our pores and become absorbed by our bodies.

. . . . .

PARASITES BREAK DOWN CELLS FOR CANCER AND A HOST OF OTHER DISEASES TO HAPPEN

. . . . .

According to Dr. Hulda Clark, Ph.D., N.D., "Most American doctors are completely unfamiliar with parasites and how they are associated with cancer, diabetes, hypoglycemia, juvenile diabetes, depression, chronic fatigue syndrome, anorexia, asthma, anemia, AIDS, learning disabilities, tumors, bulimia, colitis, epilepsy, hyperactivity syndromes, baldness, prostate trouble, arthritis, iron deficiencies, appendicitis (a favorite place for parasites), elevated white counts, Hodgkin's disease, Multiple Sclerosis (MS), psoriasis, some eczema, leukemia, lymphoma, leprosy, ulcerative colitis, low hemoglobin, poor blood quality, most bowel disorders and many more.

Symptoms of parasites in the body include: diarrhea (sometimes alternating with constipation), an ashen complexion, gas, a gurgling or growling stomach, an increase or decrease of appetite, anorexia, bulimia, an inability to gain or lose weight, low-grade fevers, coughing, hyperactivity or lethargy, grinding of teeth at night, fatigue after eating, allergies, asthma, snoring, abdominal pains, restlessness, anemia, nausea, dizziness, seizures, rectal itching, insomnia, vaginal itching, shortness of breath, intestinal bleeding, low-grade infection, blood sugar problems, colon blockages, tumor-like masses, irritability (especially around the full moon when most parasites are active), hair thinning or loss, bad breath, body odor, mucous in stools, joint pains, abdominal pains, rashes and more."

It is now known that many Americans have thousands of varieties of parasites, worms, protozoa, amoebas, bacteria, viruses and fungi. Dr. Clark states that "the presence of propyl alcohol plus parasites in the body are the cause of all cancers."

Parasites can be microscopic in size or stretch to 30 feet or longer. Under-cooked beef is a source of tapeworms. Fleas have been known to carry them as well. Hookworms can be contracted from walking barefoot on infected soil. Roundworms average six to 18 inches in length and can lay thousands of eggs each day. Other types of worms can live in liver, intestines, lungs or blood. Trichina is the tiny worm that infects pigs. Giardia is the number one water-borne disease, so beware of drinking running water in hiking areas.

Contracting parasites can be done by eating undercooked beef, through sex and casual contact, being bitten by flies, mosquitoes and eating unclean raw vegetables, drinking infected water, having close contact with dogs and other pets and simply breathing air or touching parasite-infested surfaces.

Worms can make Swiss cheese out of the organs. They can lump together and form a ball, or tumor. They can travel to the brain, heart, lungs and intestines.

Parasites have to eat, so they rob the body of nutrients. Anemia and fatigue are frequent results.

These scavengers poison the body with their toxic waste. They can be present in any disease.

The best treatment, according to Phil, is found in Dr. Clark's book: *The Cure for All Cancers & Diseases.* It takes six days to kill all the adult parasites and 90 more days to kill all the unhatched parasite eggs in the body.

Consult your homeopathic doctor and your health-food store for parasite treatment options; there are a variety on the market and to be found on line. Thorough cleansing of the body is recommended elsewhere in Phil's book as well.

. . . . .

EXPECTATIONS FOR CANCER TO OCCUR

. . . . .

One out of three persons can expect to have cancer during their lifetime and many of these cancers will return, two, three, or four times. Treatments are expensive and torturous, and many lead to other health issues. I think back to what Jim Humble said: "None of the chemicals they can give will rebuild the body or the immune system. We have to take our lives into our own hands."

The things I write in this book are from existing information found in literature that my husband gathered within the public domain of what others are doing to prevent cancer and to keep it from returning. There are a few medical and holistic doctors available if you search for them who will co-doctor. In other words, share their expertise in your treatment. There are several helpful books available if needed, such as *Step Outside the Box* by Ty Bollinger; *Cancer Doesn't Scare Me Anymore* by Dr. Lorraine Day; and *How To Cure Almost Any Cancer At Home for $5.15 a Day* by Bill Henderson with Andrew Scholberg. These could be found, if not at your local library, then I am sure online.

. . . . .

THE NATURE OF CANCER CELLS

. . . . .

Cancer cells are abnormal cells, which have been altered due to poor diet and exposure to chemicals. Some people carry genes, which facilitate certain cancers, so it's important to know your family's medical history. If for some reason that information is not available to you, medical advances now allow anyone, for a reasonable cost, to have their genetics tested. However, some individuals develop cancers through mutations that have nothing to do with their diet but may be linked to other aspects of their lives such as high levels of stress.

What we do know is that cancer cells are

opportunistic. They attack when immune defenses are weakened and health is low. Keeping a healthy diet is essential in preventing cancers. Maintaining high nutrition, eating fresh foods, and keeping a balanced level of vitamins and minerals is important. Avoiding fats, limiting red meat and low-fiber foods is equally important. Deficiencies accumulate over a long period of time, so we must be diligent with our diets, as they will eventually change the body's chemistry. Immune systems cannot function properly when the biochemistry is imbalanced.

Cancer cells feed on sugar and de-mineralized foods. Junk food and fast foods are loaded with sugars, but eliminating them from your diet is not easy if you are used to eating them. The good news is that if you can resist these foods and replace them with healthy foods, then you will no longer crave them—your body will actually reject them. Regular exercise is also important as it acts as an antioxidant to enhance body oxygen use and helps eliminate waste.

Immune systems need to be strong! Detox and cleanse your body at least twice a year. You can find fast and easy regimens for this online, such as juicing cleanses and even enemas. Be aware of possible cancer warning signals such as changes in bowel or bladder habits, a sore that does not heal, unusual bleeding or discharges, thickening or lumping in breast areas or elsewhere in the body, indigestion or difficulty in swallowing, any obvious change in a wart or mole, nagging cough or hoarseness. Remember, if you have a warning signal—don't wait—make an appointment with your doctor for a diagnosis, while a disease is in an early stage and more treatable.

It is said that cancer is a disease of the mind, body and spirit. A pro-active and positive spirit will help the cancer warrior be a survivor. Anger, un-forgiveness and bitterness put the body into a stressful and acidic environment. Learn to have a loving and forgiving spirit. Learn to relax and enjoy life. We must try to protect ourselves by learning how to lower our stress levels.

Emotional detoxification involves gaining knowledge of the ways we get ourselves sick **as well as the ways we can get ourselves well.**

- Do things that bring a sense of fulfillment, joy and purpose, that validate your worth. Make your life your own positive creation.

- Pay loving attention to yourself, by nourishing, supporting and encouraging yourself.

- Release all negative emotions, such as resentment, envy, fear, sadness and anger. Let them go. Express your feelings appropriately and forgive yourself.

· Hold positive images and goals in your mind. Picture what you truly want in your life.

· Love yourself and love others too. Make loving the purpose and primary expression in your life.

· Create fun, loving, honest relationships that allow for the expression and fulfillment of needs for intimacy and security. Try earnestly to heal wounds in past relationships.

· Make a commitment to health and well being. Develop a belief in the possibility of total health. Develop your own healing program, drawing on the support and advice of experts—without becoming enslaved to them.

. . . . .

31 Words that Stamp Out Stress

. . . . .

1. **Begin**, something that matters and don't worry about where it will take you.

2. **Imagine** that things are different with fewer struggles. Imagine living a moment of love and nourish your soul.

3. **Enjoy** being "in joy." Enjoy the freedom of dropping one major stressor in your life.

4. **Escape** as soon as you feel like a rabbit in a trap.

Escape any job that demands you pay with physical and emotional health. Escape negative people.

5. **Sigh** when no words can capture the sweet, soulful breath escaping your lips. Sigh when you want to respond but are too weary to form words.

6. **Nourish** yourself with whatever makes you feel satisfied inside and out. Know the difference between nourishing your hunger and feeding your stomach. Round out every day with the essential nourishment of peace, love, quiet and creativity.

7. **Act** *after* you've reflected and meditated, prayed and reaffirmed. Act on your instincts. Act with your own best interests at heart. Act on behalf of the young, the old or the needy.

8. **Live** in the moment as though you only have 24 hours to live the life you've always wanted. Don't just get a life, create one.

9. **Climb** higher than you ever thought you could. When you reach the top, look back and be grateful for what you've accomplished and thank those who helped you along the way.

10. **Plant** seeds of your wishes, hopes, dreams and do it in the secret garden of your heart. Be patient; they will flower in time.

11. **Embrace** a new idea, new way of looking at things. Hug someone who doesn't expect it. Hug your own wounds, your tender spots and savor the tender moments that come only once.

12. **Dare** to make waves—big ones. Dare to ask, "Why?" when everyone else is afraid to. Dare to be the youngest, the oldest, the one who says it's time for a change. Dare to lead the way.

13. **Believe** in the power of believing: happy endings or not. Believe that it matters that you don't give up when it would be easy to do so. Believe in your own instincts above anyone else's. Believe in the unbelievable if necessary.

14. **Endure** even when you think you can't stand another minute of whatever it is. Endure the heartache, the grief, the isolation. When you think you've come to the end, dig deep and endure.

15. **Rest** by turning off the computer, the phone, the lights and the noise until your soul and your body have some rest.

16. **Challenge** your body by walking, biking, bending over, stretching, dancing, and just plain moving. Challenge your mind with chess, bridge, Chaucer, chemistry, crossword puzzles. Challenge yourself to be more compassionate and genuine. Challenge yourself to become all that you can truly be. When you've reached a

new place, challenge yourself again.

17. **Reward** yourself with a chocolate kiss, an afternoon with nothing to do. Reward yourself for getting through something tough or for just being you. Write yourself a lovely note and sign it "*ME.*"

18. **Confront** your greatest fears. Confront the truth, no matter how unbelievable it may seem. Confront your inner judges and your outer critics. Confront your abuser when you're ready and with support for safety.

19. **Need** other people without being ashamed to admit it. Need help in practical-help ways and ask for it. Acknowledge your need for more love, more support, more freedom and the room to be your authentic self.

20. **Laugh** when it's too ludicrous to do anything else. Let laughter be your medicine. Share it too.

21. **Breathe** fast, slow, deep, hard until you tingle all over. When you most want to catch your breath—let it go.

22. **Connect** by sending silver strands of light and love from your heart to all those you love and even to strangers. Discover the connections that matter.

23. **Read** stories and poems, essays and your own

words in a journal. Read about people you want to emulate. Read the fine print. Read everything you've written yourself and save it.

24. **Play** hopscotch, checkers, music, with animals, with children, with friends; play tennis, pickle ball, golf, cards; play in the dirt of your garden or someone else's; even play in the mud.

25. **Clear** yourself for takeoff, pounds, mess in your attic or garage, your basement, your head or that ancient argument with yourself or someone too important to ignore. Clear up your debts and your self-defeating behavior.

26. **Slow** down and take it easy. Slow down when you drive, when you talk, when things are overwhelming. Stop running in circles. Regain control and like the turtle, live long by moving slowly.

27. **Awaken** your passion for life and awaken it in all those around you. Awaken spiritually. Find something larger than yourself to believe in. Lift yourself above the mundane. Awaken to what you've been missing.

28. **Blossom** where you're planted. Pick up a paintbrush, a hammer, a pen, a baseball, go to law school, take lessons, run for office—your time has come.

29. **Explore** where you've never gone before.

Explore a new way of living. Explore the awesome universe, your neighborhood, your friendships, your options. There's an adventure waiting.

30. **Hope** you get accepted, promoted, that you'll survive, that someone who matters actually listened to a word you said. Against all hope, continue to believe in hope.

31. **Bathe** to wash off the day or for no reason at all. Drizzle walnut oil or lavender oil onto your skin and watch it shine in the glow of a scented candle. Bathe the cracked up, dried-up places in your soul. Emerge guilt-free and dry.

. . . . .

OTHER CAUSES OF CANCER

. . . . .

Five to 10 percent of all cancers are caused by genetic mutations. By contrast, 70 to 80 percent have been linked to diet and behavioral forces.

—Karon Emmons M.D.

Dana-Farber Cancer Institute, Boston, MA

Around 1947, Dr. Virginia Livingston isolated a cancer-causing microbe, which she found in every cancer sample she analyzed, in both humans and other animals. Every person is born with this microbe, bacteria, and it stays with us until death. When our immune system is weakened by poor diet, disease, stress, or other factors, the bacteria multiplies and facilitates cancer production. Once the cancer begins to form, the bacteria release a "hormone protector that short-circuits our body's immune system." Therefore, many cancers go undetected for years. No wonder so many patients are riddled with cancers by the time they are finally diagnosed. It's important to be aware of your body's state of health. One thing you can do is order Dr. Navarro Amas's Cancer Test Kit, which can be found online. If your PSI number is over 50, then you do have concern and can begin a regime to overcome it. This number refers to the animating antibodies found in the blood stream.

If one has cancer, the priority is to slow down or stop the process of metastasis (spreading of cancer cells to other parts of the body). Metastasis and its effect on organs, blood, brain, bone marrow, etc. is what kills cancer patients. It sometimes takes years for cancer cells to turn into tumors. It is interesting that Asian men have far less prostate cancer than American men and it is believed to be due to diet.

There are basic factors that promote the development of cancer. One is weakened immunity. When people eat an unhealthy diet, not enough vegetable produce, consume too much alcohol, eat very little fish and so on, the immune system works less efficiently. This means that cancer cells can potentially slip under the radar and eventually proliferate. Another factor is that millions of Americans have sub-clinical chronic inflammation, which can lead to heart disease and cancer. Chronic inflammation can be caused by the factor of infection, such as an infected tooth, a diet low in antioxidant nutrients and even emotional stress. All these factors affect the immune system.

Cancer cells, like other cells in the body, need blood and nutrients to survive. They send out chemicals that stimulate the growth of blood vessels that carry blood to and from the cancer. This process is call angiogenesis, and it can be strongly influenced by what we eat. People who eat no more than 12 ounces of red meat weekly can reduce their overall risk for cancer by 30 percent. Red meat stimulates the release of inflammatory chemicals that inhibit apoptosis—the genetically programmed cell death that prevents uncontrolled growth.

Cancer cells cannot thrive in an oxygenated environment. Exercising daily and deep breathing help to get more oxygen down to the cellular level. Oxygen therapy—employing hyperbaric chamber procedures—is another means employed to destroy cancer cells.

It is important to understand what causes cancer, what it needs to survive and what we can do to fight it. I feel so frustrated when I pick up a newspaper and read where so and so died after a battle with cancer for an extended period of time. I think of myself, and my dear son, who really battled cancer by trying to do all the right things to kill it. Drinking wheatgrass juice, taking enemas and implants of wheatgrass juice every day, living entirely on live foods, exercising and walking every day. This truly was his battle plan, not just sitting there and letting the oncologist put poison into his body without trying to help himself.

Unfortunately, my son gave up and I truly believe he wanted to go. A Vietnam Vet in Special Forces cross-trained as a medic, he did not survive his battle with cancer. He just couldn't stay on the rigid program. He improved so much when he did this program and felt so much better, then foolishly thought he was better and went back to this original diet. He became acidic and the cancer came back with a vengeance. He then went to the oncologist and was not treated as supportively, as they knew he had been trying to do it naturally. He knew chemo was bad but by then was grasping at straws and even though the doctor told us he only had a little time to live, administered chemotherapy, which made him so ill it actually killed him. He broke out in a rash, lost his hair, and couldn't eat because all foods tasted terrible.

His last days were so sad. I said to the doctor, "You knew he was dying. Why on earth would you give him chemo knowing what it would do to him? Why didn't you explain to him what it would do to him, as we did not know? His last days could have been more peaceful." The doctor's answer was, "Well, he asked for it." I firmly feel the doctor's main purpose was to make money, as chemotherapy is incredibly lucrative. I have very little respect for that doctor and would *never* recommend him.

The cancer had metastasized all through my son's body, and the radiologist had explained that they could work with the kidneys and put a stent in but it would be painful and it is less painful to die of kidney failure than to have the stent procedure. The doctor gave him a choice and was perfectly honest with us telling us there was nothing more they could do for him. I will never know why the oncologist didn't do that and save our son from suffering so much at the end. I only wish he could have stayed on the program drinking wheatgrass juice and live foods, but I do believe it was his choice to pass on.

I, with the help of my rocket-scientist husband, who wouldn't give up on me in turn and—of course Heavenly Father—blessed me with the strength to fight my own battle with cancer. I had friends who would say, "How can you do this?" and my answer was, "If you want to live, you do it." I have several friends who have also won the battle by following the Optimum Health Institute program.

[32]

CHAPTER FOUR

EAT PROPERLY TO LOWER CANCER RISK

CHOICES WE MAKE depend upon the results of our having wellness and happiness or sickness and despair. It seems we spend the first part of our lives eating everything we want and not thinking about its nutrient value until we become ill. Then we spend the last part of our lives trying to build back our health.

When I met my husband over fifty years ago, I thought he was a hypochondriac! He ate in the best restaurants, living on steak and Lobster Thermidor. That was the thing to do back then, even though he didn't particularly want those foods, and his body rejected them by making him ill.

We are all different, no two alike, and our needs are different. We are told that some blood types require meats while others do not. My son was type

O, and according to some books, his body needed protein from animal sources. Type A, which my husband was, required vegetable proteins, and B+, which I am, could require both. It is good to know your blood type, read and review the literature to know what your body requires. I believe the evidence holds true, as my son loved meat, while my husband didn't. He didn't like chicken and was just as happy with a bowl of bean soup as he would be with a steak. I can eat everything, although I do eat very little meat. I get most of my proteins from legumes, seeds, nuts, grains, avocados, etc., and I have been quite healthy, in spite of the challenges with my heart and my bout with cancer.

We can't teach what we don't know. So many of us have grown up without giving a thought about food combinations. We have not learned that eating starch and protein at the same meal means starch is digested first and meat proteins can putrefy. The American way is to have a steak and a big baked potato for dinner! Drinking liquids with meals is not recommended as they dilute the digestive juices and make the pancreas work harder to digest our foods. But most families push liquids during meals. It's also important to chew our food thoroughly because digestion begins in the mouth. The pancreas has to work overtime when we do not give our food a head start on the way to our stomachs. An even more challenging process for our pancreatic effectiveness is burdening it with one of the most harmful substances we consume, which is white sugar!

White sugar is a dead food and robs the body of other nutrients in order to assimilate it. And no, brown sugar is not much better. I use natural sugars and stevia. Nearly all the processed foods contain amounts of white sugar. Look how many Americans suffer from diabetes, obesity and arthritic pains. One out of three will have cancer, (all sugars feed cancer like gasoline on a fire) heart problems, strokes etc. *See Chapter Seven to explore sugar concerns in detail.*

Something must be wrong with our diets. I realized a long time ago that every time I ate a lot of sweets, I would experience pain in my hands, fingers and leg cramps. When we have problems, such as arthritis pains, try to remember what you have eaten and keep track and determine which food may have caused the pain. In the summer time in Southern California, we would work in the yard on weekends and then juice a big glass of orange juice from our tree, sit on the patio and sip it. The next day my arthritic fingers would be so painful. So, from then on I would just eat the whole orange and not juice it. Then it didn't seem to trouble me. I learned that too much citrus may leach the calcium from my body. It's important to know and understand how these foods uniquely impact our bodies.

Processed foods are so bad for us. Manufacturers have taken many nutrients out and replaced them with fats, sugars, and salt to make them taste good. We were made to eat out of necessity when those hunger pains begin to rumble. It is amazing, if we eat natural foods, how quickly we become satisfied and don't over eat. God designed our bodies to require wholesome, natural food that he put here for us that would rebuild cells and keep us strong and healthy. Pizza, donuts, macaroni and cheese, white bread—all taste good, so we eat them, but these are not the foods our bodies were designed to ingest to keep us healthy.

Sadly, many people spend the beginning of their lives eating junk foods while not giving a thought about what they are eating as long as it tastes good. Then, the remainder of their lives they are trying to overcome the damage done to their bodies and attempting to regain their health.

I have a friend who tried to teach her teenage daughter about good nutrition after she read the literature and realized how important it was. She did her best to have all the healthy things that were right for her daughter, but the girl wouldn't eat it and would go out and get fattening junk food with little or no nutrients. It is so difficult to get our children to change their way of eating if it isn't stressed while they are young. Despite all the frustrations my friend went through, her daughter finally started to make healthier choices. She is now a mother of five and is very strict about their diets. Consequently, hopefully her children will do the same with their families.

. . . . .

Environmental Toxins Are Equally Bad for Us

. . . . .

I think of the dangerous chemicals used in laundry compounds, and our children sleep in blankets and clothes laundered with these compounds that may not have been completely rinsed out. Dishwashers and their chemical cleansers add to the problem with our little ones breathing the fumes, eating from "clean" dishes and crawling around on the kitchen floor, which was scrubbed with a chemical. So many things we never give a thought to are causing illnesses.

A recent EPA study concluded that the air inside American homes is up to 70 percent more polluted than outdoor air, and that toxic fumes from common household cleaners cause cancer.

I do make it a habit to turn off the air conditioning

in the summer or the heat in winter and to turn on all the fans and open the doors occasionally, for a short time, to get some fresh air.

Since no matter what preventative measures we take, we cannot escape these deadly toxins, then the best solution is to build a strong immune system by eating healthy and natural foods, so our bodies can fight illnesses. This is something my husband and I both did regularly using Dr. Schulze's incredible natural cleansing program. If one has a cholesterol problem it has been reported that keeping the liver cleansed will also help cholesterol levels to remain within a normal range.

In an introduction to cleansing, Phil noted, "In years past, it has been stated that cleanliness is next to Godliness. Today, we live in a world that has environmental pollution greater than at any time in the history of man." John Robbins in one of his books entitled *Diet for a New America*, and others of his writings, describes the polluted environment we live in and its effect on the foods we eat and what we must do to have optimum health.

He explained how toxins enter our bodies and failure to eliminate these toxins causes build up in various parts of the body such as hips, knees, and joints, plus the colon area. The movable parts of our body are cleansed and flushed daily if we drink 8 to 10 glasses of distilled, or purified water and do plenty of exercise. A build-up of toxins in the colon causes auto-toxicity wherein the toxins enter the bloodstream and travel to various parts of the body causing contamination, illness and various health maladies. Elimination of toxic waste material from the colon is accomplished by having at least one bowel movement daily. At best we should have a bowel movement an hour after each meal. Of course, all these factors have to do with the food we eat, how it is grown, prepared and combined with other foods.

I try to keep a jar of sauerkraut that I make myself with kelp—instead of so much salt—in the refrigerator and have a tablespoon with one of my daily meals. Any fermented product such as this will help keep healthy bacteria in the colon, doing the job they should. Probiotics are very important.

Over the period of many years, the colon and various sub-systems of the body become sluggish and under perform because of age and toxicity. These sub-systems such as the liver, gallbladder, kidneys, bladder, blood as well as the colon need to be cleansed to return them to their full operating performance levels.

Without realizing it, many people suffer from a buildup of intestinal parasites and heavy metals. Most family doctors are not trained in basic or advanced nutritional methods and therefore do not recommend to their patients the need for internal cleansing for their bodies. Dr. Schulze, who was a student of the well-known naturopathic healer of this era, John R. Christopher, has helped our family by providing cleansing programs that have helped to keep our family healthy. The old adage, one can lead a horse to water but you can't make it drink, is true with our families. We can teach correct principals but it is up to each of us what we do with that knowledge.

I have read that there is a protective mantel on our skin that helps prevent bacteria from entering our bodies. I often think about how our modern-day civilization has so many illnesses. Besides all of the chemicals in our soil, water and food; poor eating and other unhealthy habits, the natural protection of our skin may be compromised these days.

My mother taught us that cleanliness was next to Godliness and she made certain we washed our hands before we could eat. I remember when it was time for us to go to bed she would have us go out to the stream of water that ran through our yard, because we didn't have running water in our house back in thirties. We loved to go barefoot all day, so she would have us wash our feet in the stream before going to bed. We took a sponge bath during the week, but Saturday night was bath night when she heated pots of water on the wood-burning stove. Dad brought in the big metal bathtub and placed it on the floor next to the stove so we would be warm. They put a ring of chairs facing backward around the tub and draped blankets over the chairs for privacy. We all took our baths in order: first my sister and I, and then our brothers. We were all snuggly tucked into bed in our clean underwear and jammies.

I know I bathed my children every night before they went to bed and bath time was so much fun for them. These days, we tend to shower every night, sometimes more often during the day after sports activities or before going to dressy events. Are we washing that protective skin mantel off? I wonder if perhaps this contributes to our children having health problems.

. . . . .

For Optimum Health, Avoid Plastic Utensils and Microwave Use

. . . . .

Johns Hopkins' research has warned us to not freeze plastic bottles with water in them as this releases dioxin from the plastic. We are told that we should not drink ice water, as it shocks the spleen, and that the best water for the body is water at room temperature. Also, do not use plastic containers in a microwave. In fact, we are told to stop using microwaves altogether as they are sterilizers and kill all enzymes in the food. When cooking with a microwave we are giving our bodies worthless food.

Recently, Dr. Edward Fujimoto, Wellness Program Manager at Castle Hospital, was on a TV program to explain the health hazard of plastic. He said how bad dioxins are for us and that we should not heat our foods in the microwave using plastic containers or plastic wrap. This especially applies to foods that contain fat. He said that the combination of fat and the heat and plastics releases dioxin into the food and ultimately into the cells of the body. Instead, he recommends, if you must use the microwave, use glass, such as Corning Ware, Pyrex or ceramic containers for heating food. TV dinners, instant ramen and soups, etc., should be removed from the purchase container and heated in tempered glass. Most fast-food establishments have moved away from the use of foam containers to paper. (The paper source and preservative chemicals may be in question, however.)

The Toxic Chemicals in Our Homes Manufacturers Aren't Telling Us About

Phil passed on the information to his classes that several every-day consumer products are made with toxic chemical ingredients that are nowhere to be found on the package label.

He quoted a study I cannot find the source for, but the information is worth sharing with our readers:

Forty household products such as hair coloring, lipstick, paints, cleaners, detergents and the like were tested for toxic-chemical content. Out of the 40 products, evidence for the following chemicals was discovered in 34 of them: glycols, organic solvents and phthalates did not appear on the labels.

Although the study didn't test at what level these chemicals were harmful to people, they did find that they could contribute to impacting the nervous system, reproductive system and cause or exacerbate other health issues in a person's body.

Researchers stated the most common toxic chemicals that could be inhaled from household products are chlorine, toluene, xylene, methyl, ethyl ketone and n-hexane, a danger for children to breathe.

Most pressed-wood furniture contains formaldehyde, which can cause allergic reactions and long-term is a known carcinogen. Whenever possible purchase solid-wood furniture.

The same concerns are true for Teflon nonstick-coated cooking pans, which release toxic particles when heated above 500°. Use ceramic, cast-iron or stainless-steel utensils to ensure your safety.

Keeping health and safety in mind, whenever possible think of and select alternatives to commercially available chemical products.

For example, a formula of natural ingredients for controlling cockroaches and ants in the home is a non-toxic alternative to commercial insect repellent or "killer" sprays.

Powdered sugar and borax combined in equal parts and sprinkled where these pests crawl is effective and harmless to pets and people.

Taking off your shoes before entering your home is recommended because they track in lawn chemicals and heavy metals that are then deposited in your carpets and on other floor surfaces. They can be inhaled and are of course a direct danger to little children crawling on the floor.

A tip I share is a habit Phil and I used to minimize toxic buildup in a heated car. The upholstery and plastic surfaces in a car can heat up to well above 120°–180° or more—in a closed car sitting in a sunny parking lot. All of those materials contain toxic ingredients. Upon returning to a hot car, enter and leave the car doors open and windows down. With the air conditioner on, allow surfaces to return to a lower temperature. Let the fumes dissipate before closing up the car. If the steering wheel is too hot to handle, don't sit there and breathe chemical emissions, even cooled cars with the air conditioners on are harmful.

. . . . .

CELL PHONES EMIT RADIATION IN OUR HOMES AND CARS

. . . . .

Not only should we clean our cellphones with alcohol wipes to kill germs as dangerous as E. coli bacteria, we need to become more aware of the danger in radiation emitted by them.

To reduce radiation risk, put your cell on speaker phone to talk and keep it away from your body between calls. Do not leave it near your bed. Avoid long conversations when the signal is weak, which forces the phone to work at a higher power.

The danger is greatest to youth whose brains are still developing. Sufficient long-term study has not been forthcoming to clarify the degree of impairments with cell phone use, but researchers in neurological labs are deeply concerned about the issue of cell-phone use long-term.

. . . . .

Is Tuna Fish Safe or Is Mercury a Genuine Hazard?

. . . . .

Mercury emissions from power plants around the globe settle into bodies of water where large fish consume small fish. Tuna and swordfish, very large fish, have significant buildup of mercury and when people consume them, their bodies store this deadly toxin, which can affect the body's neurological system.

Studies have linked mercury to learning impairment in children. Almost 35 percent of the mercury consumed in the U.S. comes from tuna. The FDA advises nursing mothers and women who are pregnant or may become pregnant should eat no more than 12 ounces of chunk light tuna a week and no more than 6 ounces of solid-white albacore, which is higher in mercury.

The maximum mercury consumption the EPA said was safe is one microgram a day for each 22 pounds of body weight. If a 130-pound woman ate as much albacore as the federal advisory allows, she would exceed that level by 40 percent.

Of course, we know tuna is high in Omega-3 fatty acids, which—minus mercury—are good for the body. However, is it worth the risk? Canned tuna is high in mercury. That fact is established.

CHAPTER FIVE

THE BENEFITS OF VEGETARIANISM IN COMBATTING CANCER

Nothing will benefit human health and increase the chances of the survival of life on earth as much as the evolution of a vegetarian diet.
—Albert Einstein

CANCER CELLS HAVE a tough protein covering. By refraining from or eating less meat it frees more enzymes to attack the protein walls of cancer cells and allows the body's killer cells to destroy the cancer cells.

The main categories of cancer include:

- **carcinoma**—cancer that begins in the skin or in tissues that line or cover internal organs.

- **Sarcoma**—cancer that begins in bone, cartilage, fat, muscle, blood vessels, or other connective or supportive tissue.

- **Leukemia**—cancer that starts in blood-forming tissue such as the bone marrow and causes large numbers of abnormal blood cells to be produced and to enter the blood stream.

· **Lymphoma** and **myeloma**—cancers that begin in the cells of the immune system.

· **Central nervous system cancers**—cancers that begin in the tissues of the brain and spinal cord.

For definitions of other cancer-related terms, consult National Cancer Institute (NCI's) Dictionary of Cancer Terms.

Do check for information in your local libraries. We have our Regional Medical Center here in St. George that is very informative. There is Huntsman (IHC) Cancer Center, our local library, and Pioneer Utah Credible Online Research Library, which is supported by taxpayer's funds and is cost free to the public, Huntsman Cancer Learning Center in Salt Lake City, Utah which contains over 3,300 books, audiotapes, CDs, DVDs and CD-ROMs (Most items are available for checkout without charge.) To borrow books for three weeks and Audio-visual available for 10 days call 1-800-581-6365 or 1-888-424-2100, Monday through Friday 8 A.M. to 4 P.M. Do some research about the topics you are interested in knowing more about in this book, and see what information is available to improve your health and that of your family members.

. . . . .

Protein Sources to Maintain Optimum Health as a Vegetarian

. . . . .

Diet is so very important. We should become aware of our nutritional needs in order to stay healthy. Some people wonder if they attempt to maintain a mostly vegetarian diet, will they still get the amount of protein needed to be healthy. That is a concern we must be aware of.

Some dear friends of Phil's and mine had a daughter who decided to become a vegetarian and wouldn't touch meat to 'save the world,' or so she said. Her health declined, as she wasn't knowledgeable, didn't eat properly and indulged in a lot of junk food, as opposed to balancing her diet with sufficient protein.

Actually, in our society today, people are getting too much protein—not too little. In checking with the Vegetarian Society of Utah, (VSU) we learn that one can get enough protein from whole wheat bread, oatmeal, beans, corn, peas, mushrooms, avocado, broccoli, seeds, and nuts. Almost every food contains protein. Protein is very important and necessary for the body's growth, repair, and maintenance. Women need only about 44 grams of protein per day, less than 2 oz.; and men require about 56 grams (about 2 oz.). The average American eats about 90 grams of protein per day.

We should be aware that excess *animal-sourced* protein overworks the liver and kidneys and may cause problems with other organs of the body. The bones can lose calcium from too much protein, leading to osteoporosis, which cannot be corrected by eating a lot of calcium-rich foods.

I have a very dear friend, who along with her husband, ate a lot of animal products, such as meat and milk products. I tried to tell her what I had learned about not doing that when I was fighting cancer. She wouldn't listen. Today, she is crippled from osteoporosis, and it breaks my heart. Another friend who was a chef, lived on steak and other fine cuts of meat. He died from heart problems way too young.

Plant protein is made up of the same building blocks, called "amino acids," as animal protein. The body doesn't know the difference. We are told that our bodies will build proteins from the amino acids present in vegetables, grains, and legumes. I have read where some of our best world athletes are vegetarians. Athletes require a little more protein than the average person. They certainly need more calories because of their energy output, and these calories can come from carbohydrates not protein.

Sources of protein sufficient to keep us healthy are: potatoes, beans, (kidney, lima, black, pinto, garbanzo (chickpeas), whole-wheat bread, rice, broccoli, spinach, almonds, peas, tofu, almond milk, lentils, kale, oatmeal, corn, mushrooms, Tempeh Seitan, legumes, peanuts, quinoa, chia seeds, walnuts, almonds, pecans, sunflower seeds, cashews, brown rice, veggie burgers, Boca Burgers™, etc. Do a search on Google and find more on the Internet. The Recommended Dietary Allowance (RDA) for protein, for the average sedentary adult, is only 0.4 grams per pound of body weight. To find out your average individual need, simply perform the following calculation: Body weight (in pounds) x 0.4 = recommended protein intake per day. Example: A 130-pound person needs about 52 grams of protein per day.

The American Dietetic Association reports: "Scientific data suggests positive relationships between a vegetarian diet and reduced risk for several chronic degenerative diseases and conditions including: obesity, coronary-artery disease, hypertension, diabetes, mellitus, and some types of cancer. Do check out additional resources for information, such as: www.thechinastudy.com, www.veganhealth.org/articles/protein, www.pcrm. org/health/veginfo/protein.html.

The Vegetarian Society of Utah said that a startling discovery had been found and reported in T. Colin Campbell, Ph.D.'s, book *The China Study* that animal protein is a key-player in producing many forms of cancer. That in 27 years of research, which was peer reviewed in the best scientific journals, results conclusively showed that "low-protein diets inhibited the initiation of cancer by aflatoxin, a toxic carcinogen. In fact, dietary protein proved to be so powerful in its effect that we could turn on and turn off cancer growth simply by changing the level of protein consumed."

An analysis of the types of protein that promoted cancer confirmed, that "Casein, which makes up 87 percent of cow's milk protein, promoted all stages of the cancer process."

Whereas "safe protein, which did not promote cancer, was found to be plant-based protein." They said in laboratory tests, rats were divided into two groups. Both groups were subjected to the same dosage of the toxin carcinogen (aflatoxin) that promotes cancer. One group was fed a 20 percent animal protein diet; the other group was fed a 5 percent animal protein diet. After 100 weeks, all that were fed the 20 percent had died while the ones consuming 5 percent were still alive and well.

The average American consumes way too much protein. The test showed that nutrients from animal-based foods increased tumor development, while nutrients from plant-based foods decreased tumor development (see pg. 53 *The China Study*).

Cooked foods could include beans soaked overnight, sprouted, and cooked. Fresh vegetables and vegetable juice provide live enzymes that are easily absorbed and reach down to cellular levels within a few minutes to nourish and enhance growth of healthy cells. To obtain live enzymes for building healthy cells, try eating a diet of 80 percent raw vegetables and fruit.

As we know, enzymes are destroyed when cooked over 104° F or 40° C. For optimum health as a vegetarian, the emphasis for food quality should be organic raw fruits, vegetables, nuts, and seeds.

FOODS TO SUPPORT OPTIMUM HEALTH

FOOD IS OUR BEST MEDICINE—good food, that is. The fresher, the better! Even organic fruits and vegetables can lose up to 50 percent of their nutrients in just 3 days, so visit your garden to pick and your local market to select as often as possible. Rinse them in hot water and they will keep better. Millions of people from children to older adults are not consuming the essential nutrients to maintain optimal health. As stated previously, many of the foods we buy from grocery stores increase our risk for diseases as serious as cancer, heart issues, and stroke.

You don't have to be poor or skinny to be malnourished in today's world. Many people are seriously deficient in nutrients and are vulnerable to disease and premature aging. Proper diets may help us avoid many of these illnesses.

Consider what you consume daily. Many of us wake in the morning, drink a cup of coffee with or without sugars, possibly eat a piece of toast, and then run off to work. Lunch may be a fast-food cheeseburger or taco and for dinner a pizza. Some may even gulp down a handful of supplements to account for their missed vitamin intake. However, many of these supplements may be toxic! Read labels carefully and consult health experts.

In nature, everything is balanced, so our bodies utilize the food intake with all the associated food factors to help assimilate it. Bodies then know what they need to promote cell division and healing. If given proper food, the cells are strong and healthy. If given improper foods, the cells are weak and easily succumb to illnesses.

Every minute, every hour, every day, there is a fierce battle raging inside our bodies. We are under constant attack from infectious bacteria, viruses, parasites, and an army of unfriendly microbes who want to make our bodies their permanent home. Our immune system is our defense against this onslaught. Once our body is weakened from improper diet, the viruses, fungi, and cancers take over. We must fight to keep our immune systems well maintained.

Because nutrition is vital to health, schools should teach mandatory nutritional health courses.

I think on this often since I left the farm. Where once I had unlimited access to fresh vegetables, raw milk, and organic meats, I suddenly found delicious, artificial foods of the typical American: sodas, candies, and white bread. I didn't have a clue about what damage I was doing to my body, nor does any young person these days. Everything tasted wonderful! So I ate anything I wanted without the knowledge to support my own healthy eating.

My husband Phil tried to help others with what we have learned. I'm doing my best to work from his lecture notes to share with our readers how to achieve and maintain optimum health.

Optimum health requires optimum nutrition; our modern diet is not cutting it. Having a proper diet may seem difficult and time-consuming. Time most of us can't recuperate, but there are many delicious ways to enhance our diets without adding too much more time to our daily routine.

It is sad that more people won't take control of their lives. Many of us seem to overeat and eat without thinking of nutrient value. They say that people who are deficient in magnesium are most likely to experience sudden cardiac arrest. This mineral prevents blood clots, dilates blood vessels, and can also stop the development of dangerous heart irregularities. And important for bones and body tissue.

Magnesium-rich foods are nuts and seeds. Pecans are very high in magnesium, and seeds— pumpkin seeds especially, dark rich chocolate, green leafy vegetables, whole grains, bananas, avocados and fish.

LIQUIDS

Avoid coffee, tea, and alcohol. The former two have high amounts of caffeine. Green tea is a better alternative and has cancer-fighting properties. Water is best to drink purified or filtered to avoid known toxins and heavy metals in tap water.

SOY

Dr. David Servan-Schreiber, M.D., Ph.D., University of Pittsburgh School of Medicine recommends that women who are cancer free should have three servings of soy per week. AVOID soy if you are concerned that estrogen-like compounds in soy might promote tumor growth in women who have a type of breast cancer that is activated by estrogen's effects.

According to John A. McDougall, M.D., author of The McDougall Program, the myth is: Tofu is a perfectly healthy meat and dairy substitute. The fact is: People in search of better health often replace meat and dairy products with soybeans and their derivatives such as tofu, soy cheese, soy milk, miso and tempeh. They contain far too much fat for regular use. Tofu is a high-fat and low-fiber food. Use these soy foods as special treats only.

MUSHROOMS

Asian mushrooms, such as shitake, maitake, and enokitake, are available in most supermarkets and as a group are one of the most potent immune system stimulants. Among people who eat a lot of these mushrooms, the rate of stomach cancer is 50 percent lower than it is among those who don't eat them. One to two-cup servings weekly seemed to be effective. Dr. Servan-Schreiber also tells us that blue berries and blackberries contain elegiac acid, which inhibits angiogenesis. Perhaps one-half cup per day is sufficient.

WHEATGRASS

Let's look at the benefits of consuming wheatgrass juice for those who are ill and wish to do something healthy to be well and happy again and who will take the time to help themselves. Phil and I had a rack in the laundry room near a window for sunlight with a drainage pan underneath and kept wheatgrass growing continually.

We juiced it every day and drank 2 ounces of

this vibrant, rich in green chlorophyll life-giving nutrient. It is literally condensed sunlight energy. It is one of the most nutritionally potent healing agents on the planet. The taste isn't that good but the results I had were amazing. To make wheatgrass more palatable, add a dash of cinnamon.

It is so simple to grow.

Get trays from the nursery, line with black print newspapers (no color, as the dye is toxic) and add about 1 inch of potting soil. Soak red winter wheat overnight in purified water, drain and spread over the soil and cover with about 8 layers of wet newspaper. Keep this damp all the time until you see a little sprout appearing. Remove the newspaper, and water as needed. It takes 7 days to reach about 7 inches in height and is then ready to be cut and juiced. In the summer, you can do this outside—but not in full sun.

Research history has determined that wheatgrass was identified as the finest grass food of all after a series of intensive agricultural research studies spearheaded by Dr. Charles Schnozzle and assisted by Dr. George Kohler, Dr. Richard Graham, Conrad A. Evehjem and E. B. Hart in the 1930s, '40s and '50s. They performed direct comparisons of wheatgrass against other well-regarded vegetables including spinach, broccoli and alfalfa.

Further research showed that wheatgrass

contains a broad spectrum of vitamins, minerals, antioxidants, amino acids, essential fatty acids and enzymes.

Ann Wigmore, independent of the agricultural research studies above told us when prisoners in a concentration camp were almost starving on the meager diet given them—one family found bunches of grass they chewed for sustenance. That family stayed healthier than other prisoners and survived.

Wigmore was the founder of the Hippocrates Health Institute in Boston and worked with thousands of people over the years to help them get well. Now we have Optimum Health Institute of San Diego, which she and Rachel founded, that has helped so many of us find our way back to health. They don't claim to cure ailments and diseases, only teach how to take care of our bodies so that our bodies will heal themselves. I attended the one in Lemon Grove, California.

CHOCOLATE

For chocolate lovers, apparently one ounce of dark chocolate contains twice as many polyphenols as a glass of red wine and almost as much as a cup of green tea. It should be 70 percent cocoa. The lighter chocolate does not contain this ingredient.

Whether we have cancer, heart problems or other ailments, we should be aware of the healing power of flax and add this to our family's diet as this is one of the richest source of Omega-3 and there is no after taste as with fish oil products and it is more affordable. If you prefer to use the Flax oil it has a delicious nutty flavor, making it easy to incorporate into your diet as a salad dressing, stirred into oatmeal, mixed into yogurt or combined with a blender smoothie. Many times, I have soaked flax seed overnight in purified water and added it to my smoothies. My family never knew that it was in there.

Several studies have shown that our typical Omega -3 level in our bodies is 80 percent below normal. Dr. Budwig's work has confirmed that processed foods, margarine, etc. that contain "hydrogenated" fat causes this drop in Omega-3 levels. The flaxseed oil, when mixed with organic cottage cheese or yogurt restores that balance.

Dr. Williams, health guru, urges us to drastically increase our intake of Omega-3 fatty acids, which are most critical for our cardiovascular system, cholesterol, blood pressure, brain function, immune system, joints, and just about every other system in our bodies.

<u>Turmeric, The Queen of the Spices</u>

One of the simplest ways to prevent or treat cancer could be the use of the common Asian plant known as turmeric (*Zingiberaceae*). This ginger-like spice, which has been used in medicine for over 4,000 years!, is used in a variety of Asian foods from savory to sweet and can be eaten raw, cooked, or ground into a fine powder.

Aside from its substantial contribution of iron, potassium, vitamins C and B, calcium, manganese, zinc, and fiber, it may also be crucial in the prevention and reduction of most cancers due to its effects on the immune system.

Turmeric is brimming with antioxidants five to eight times more potent than vitamins and three times more potent than grape seed or pine bark extract. It supports brain and cardiac health as well as joint and digestive health. Additionally, Dr. David Servan-Schreiber suggests turmeric can be used as an anti-inflammatory, unlike any other food.

This spice contains curcumin, which inhibits the growth of a variety of cancers, and promotes the death of cancer cells. Asian countries are often associated with low rates of cancer. It isn't much of a leap to assume turmeric may be part of the secret! In India, most people consume an average of 1/4 tsp to 1/2 tsp of the spice every day. This may have to do with the 1/8 as many lung cancers as those of us in Western countries (e.g., the United States) even when accounting for ages of the people involved in studies. Also, these turmeric consumers have 1/9 as many colon cancers and 1/5 as many breast cancers compared to their Western counterparts.

Turmeric is inexpensive and relatively easy to come by. However, if it isn't pure, it can do more harm than good. Be diligent in selecting brands which are independently certified organic for quality and do not contain chalk or artificial color.

A water test for chalk powder in turmeric is easy and quick: In a clear glass of warm water, drop 1 teaspoon of turmeric powder on its surface. The water will become cloudy with sediments settling to the bottom. After 20 minutes, if there is no chalk, all sediments will have settled to the bottom and the water will be clear yellow. Of course, if the water is cloudy, chalk is present.

Artificial colors are more worrisome. To discover their presence in the turmeric product, mix 1/2 teaspoon turmeric powder with 4 teaspoons of water to which a few drops of strong household vinegar (white) has been added. If the water turns pink, purple or violet, artificial yellow is present, dangerous and cancer causing in significant amounts.

For the Turmeric Golden Milk recipe, refer to

Chapter 16, page 181. Simply add 1/2 teaspoon of turmeric powder into your hot green tea with a splash of organic honey for an immunity boost to start your day. For lunch, try adding a bit of turmeric paste to your favorite salad dressing! You can add it to any of your favorite foods from smoothies to curries to soups. *The recipe for Turmeric Paste is in the Chapter 16 as well.*

CHAPTER SEVEN

SUGAR CAUTIONS

I F PARENTS ONLY REALIZED how bad soda drinks are for children's health, they would never buy and bring them home or order them in a restaurant.

Sugar is addictive. If one can refrain from eating anything with sugar in it, over time the body will reject it. I know when I was fighting cancer and lived on all live foods, etc. even to look at a piece of cake made me feel ill. However, pie was a different story, as I grew up with the best homemade pies in the world that my little mother would bake for us. I still love pie and eat it occasionally if I make it myself with my own recipe, using raw sugar and stevia. But they are never as good as I remember my mother's were.

According to Langreth and Stanford's reporting

of Bloomberg findings, foods, snacks and beverages sweetened with sugar and high fructose corn syrup are addictive, and are probably the major cause of rampant obesity in children and adults. Hopefully the likely consumer-safety battle on the horizon will match the anti-smoking movement a generation ago.

We had a friend whose daughter had to be hospitalized for kidney failure. It was discovered that she had been drinking several cola drinks every day. An article written by Mike Stobbs, an AP medical writer, stated that half of Americans drink a soda daily and some are downing a lot more. One in 20 people drink the equivalent of more than four cans each day. Even though health officials say sweetened beverages should be limited to less than half a can, many refuse to break the habit. Stobbs notes that sweetened drinks have been linked to the U.S. explosion in obesity and related medical problems. Health officials have been urging people to cut back on soda/cola drinks for years. Some officials have proposed an extra soda tax and many schools have stopped selling soda or artificial juices.

If blood sugar is getting low, stevia is a safe sweetener that can be used (there is a section to follow on this sugar substitute), as can an occasional Granny Smith apple or a tiny amount of Manuka honey or molasses. There are dangers in using sugar substitutes such as: NutraSweet, Equal, Splenda, Aspartame, etc. It is best not to use table salt. One may use Bragg's liquid amino or a little sea salt, Himalayan preferred.

Milk can cause the body to produce mucus, especially in the gastro-intestinal tract. Cancer feeds on mucus. By cutting out milk and substituting unsweetened almond, or coconut milk, cancer cells are being starved. (Note: Soy milk is high in estrogen, so if you do not have high estrogen receptors, do not use it because estrogen can activate cancer.)

As noted above by Stobbs in the AP report on the CDC findings that about half the population drinks a sugared beverage each day; how that breaks out is interesting. Males consume more than females, with teenage boys leading the pack.

· · · · ·

THE DIET DRINK MYTH

· · · · ·

I recently read an article from *Trends* asking whether zero-calorie drinks make you gain weight. It stated that researchers tracked 474 older adults for nearly a decade and found that the waistlines of diet-soda drinkers expanded remarkably more than those of people who avoided these drinks.

In fact, those who drank two or more diet sodas

daily saw their waistlines expand by an average of 4.7 centimeters (about 2 inches). The crucial factor is artificial sweeteners such as aspartame and Sucralose. They contain virtually no calories but have negative health effects, as supported by researcher Helen Hazuda, Ph.D. of the University of Texas Health Science Center. She is quoted as saying, "Artificial sweeteners are about 180 times sweeter than regular sugar", which can make you crave (and eat) sweeter and high-fat foods.

. . . . .

Limit Soda Beverages

. . . . .

Dr. Hazuda recommends avoiding, or if you can't, at least limit soda drinks to one per week. Try to substitute teas or fresh fruit juice as healthier alternatives.

From *Healthwise*, we are told by Nancy Appleton, Ph.D., that bottled fruit juice is almost as bad as soft drinks because of the added sugar, which includes all the sugar that isn't naturally present in foods. A twelve-ounce can of Pepsi has about 10 teaspoons of sugar. Most soft drinks have a similar amount of sugar as do bottled teas and sports drinks. However, the diet forms of these sodas contain, in addition to sugar, phosphoric acid (which disrupts mineral balance), if not high fructose corn syrup (a form of sugar that may increase the risk for metabolic syndrome); they contain chemical sweetener replacements and caffeine (which can cause heart palpitations and insomnia).

Dr. Appleton also cautions that even real fruit juice, including fresh apple, grape and orange juice contains about 10 teaspoons of natural sugar to every glass. Natural juice sugar upsets your body chemistry in the same way that added sugar does. So, it is best to eat the whole fruit, not just to juice it and dispose of the pulp and rind. Our bodies weren't designed to process much sweetness. Excess sugar breaks down the process of homeostasis, the body's ability to maintain a healthy chemical balance.

What this can lead to is calcium depletion because sugar acidifies the blood. The body attempts to restore a normal state of alkalinity by removing calcium from the bones. This increases blood levels of calcium while decreasing bone levels. The result is a higher risk for bone fractures and osteoporosis, along with an increased risk for cardiovascular disease from arterial calcification.

Sugar-caused blood acidity can also lead to auto-immune diseases. Mineral imbalances caused by excess sugar and phosphoric acid, impair the normal functions of enzymes, including digestive enzymes. When these can't function, protein molecules from incompletely digested foods can pass through the intestine and into the bloodstream. These "foreign" molecules then are attacked by the immune system. This condition is known as 'leaky gut syndrome'. This condition can increase the risk for and/or severity of lupus, rheumatoid arthritis and other autoimmune diseases.

Swedish researchers sent food questionnaires to nearly 80,000 men and women. They found that those who consumed the most sugar, particularly from soft drinks were significantly more likely to have pancreatic cancer. Dr. Nancy Appleton's book *Lick the Sugar Habit* explains the 78 ways sugar can ruin your health and would be a good place to start changing habits related to sugar in foods as well as drinks.

. . . . .

ASPARTAME AND SUCRALOSE, THE TOXIC SUGAR REPLACEMENTS

. . . . .

NOTE: Aspartame is the technical name for the brand names NutraSweet, Equal, Spoonful, and Equal Measure. It's dangerous stuff.

The following list of several Internet articles and reports on (NutraSweet) Aspartame and (Sucralose) Splenda should prove useful to readers.

From *Shirley's Wellness Café*, "Holistic Health Care for People and Animals" we read the bitter truth about Aspartame. It appears to have a profound effect on mood and cognition. Depressed mood, anxiety, dizziness, panic attacks, nausea, irritability, impairment of memory and concentration as said by Ralph Walton, M.D. i.e. "We have known for years that when aspartame is ingested with a carbohydrate-rich meal the usual physiologic increase in tryptophan is blocked, while brain phenylalanine and tyrosine concentrations are increased. These changes in amino-acid blocked neurotransmitter precursors could, I believe, alter indoleamine/catecholamine balance, and thus have a profound effect on mood and cognition. And as noted above. depressed mood, anxiety, dizziness, panic attacks, nausea, irritability, impairment of memory and concentration.

The testing of Sucralose (Splenda) reveals that it can cause up to 40 percent shrinkage of the thymus: a gland that is the very foundation of our immune system. Sucralose also causes swelling of the liver and kidneys, and calcification of the kidney. Dr. Janet Starr Hull suggests if you experience kidney pain, cramping or an irritated bladder after using Sucralose—stop using it immediately.

Dr. H. J. Roberts, M.D. noted that he had observed   severe   intellectual   deterioration associated with the use of aspartame products. Usually manifested as great difficulty in reading and writing, obvious problems with memory, and grossly impaired orientation to time, place and person. Many reactions to aspartame were very serious including seizures and death. Other reactions the report included were: headaches/migraines, dizziness, joint pain, nausea, numbness, muscle spasms, weight gain, rashes, depression, fatigue, irritability, tachycardia, insomnia, vision loss, hearing loss, heart palpitations, breathing difficulties, anxiety attacks, slurred speech, loss of taste, tinnitus, vertigo, and memory loss.

Doctor Roberts also declared Aspartame Disease to be a global plague. Roberts has now published a medical text titled: *Aspartame Disease; an Ignored Epidemic*.

James Bowen, M.D. declared "Lying and deceit on the artificial sweetener issue has been the FDA's modus operandi ever since Donald Rumsfeld broke everything decent in the US government to put aspartame on the market as a "contract on humanity". Either they have done but little testing of Sucralose, or they are so afraid of what the public would think of Sucralose, and the government if the public but knew what was going on, that they will not tell us! *Because*: "We have been told nothing about the extensive studies which would have to have been done if very reasonable and scientifically sound FDA rules had been followed."

Coca-Cola, Pepsi, and NutraSweet were sued in California on April 6, 2004. Lawsuits were filed in three separate California courts against twelve companies who either produce or use the artificial sweetener aspartame as a sugar substitute in their products. The suits were filed in Shasta, Sonoma and Butte counties, California.

"Racketeering Charges Filed Against Companies for Manufacturing and Marketing Toxic Aspartame" is a headline of note. The National Justice League filed a $350 million class-action lawsuit on September 15, 2004 in San Francisco, California, in Federal District Court against NutraSweet, Monsanto, The American Diabetes Association and Dr. Robert H. Moser, Former FDA commissioner.

The FDA has received over 5,500 complaints against aspartame (NutraSweet), which was legalized amid controversy regarding the capacity of this substance to alter brain hormone balances; some 9 percent of the complaints today involve serious neurological effects, including seizures. Do read: *Sweet Poison: How the World's Most Popular Artificial Sweetener Is killing Us*, by Janet Starr Hull. This is a must-read for anyone who is still consuming food or drinks containing aspartame.

Systemic lupus has become almost as rampant as multiple sclerosis, especially with Diet Coke and Diet Pepsi drinkers. When the temperature of Aspartame exceeds 86° F, the wood alcohol in it converts to formaldehyde and then to formic acid, which in turn causes metabolic acidosis. Formic acid is the poison found in stinging fire ants. Methanol toxicity is a death sentence.

We must become knowledgeable of what we are putting into our bodies. Remember that James Bowen, M.D. said, "Splenda is not splendid!"

Johnson and Johnson's McNeil Nutritionals, who make Splenda have been slapped with a number of lawsuits accusing them of falsely advertising Splenda and deceiving buyers into believing it is a natural product. They make the statement: "Splenda, No Calorie Sweetener, is made from sugar so it tastes like sugar." Taste does not make it safe.

. . . . .

Stevia: a Safe, Natural Sweetener

. . . . .

So what is the answer to how we can replace as much sweetener as we need to in order to stay healthy? Do become knowledgeable about how stevia is a safe natural alternative to sugar and all sugar substitutes. Stevia is a plant. I grow it in my garden and harvest the leaves and put them in my iced-mint tea. It is a member of the Chrysanthemum family and grows wild in South America. It has been safely used for centuries.

The Japanese consume the greatest amount of stevia as artificial sweeteners are banned in Japan! Smart people. The plant found in the wild is very different from the sweetener most of us are using. Stevia, derived from the leaf of the Paraguayan herb and available as a starter plant for your garden, is produced as a powder or in liquid form and is approximately 300 times sweeter than sugar. Even though these forms are not natural stevia, they are supposedly better than sugar. However, use it sparingly. It is also diluted from its high potency and can be purchased in liquid form. Apparently it is the stevioside that the stevia plant contains that has the health benefits. The processed stevia has not been tested in regard to its capacity to help alleviate health problems.

Stevia, we are told, is still one of the best options when replacing sugar in one's diet. It is beneficial for at least two reasons: potential medical properties that may help with healing and avoiding sugar that causes so many health problems.

When buying stevia we are told to buy organic, with no unnatural additives, and to avoid added alcohol.

Stevia has been shown to increase energy and aid in digestion by stimulating the pancreas. Research has shown that stevia controls blood-sugar levels used by people with hypoglycemia and diabetes. No research has ever found stevia to be harmful. The FDA allows stevia to be sold as a nutritional supplement and not as a sweetener. It is available in local health-food stores and online. For more information, contact: Omega Nutrition 1-800-661-3529. Search online and read more about this natural sweetener.

I do use, occasionally, some raw sugar, honey or pure maple syrup, but as I noted before I substitute stevia (Stevia by brand name) for much of the raw sugar. Your family will never know the difference and you will be helping them to stay healthier.

THE STEVIA EQUIVALENT CHART

Sugar	Equivalent Stevia *Powder*	Equivalent Stevia *Liquid*
1 cup	1 tsp	1 tsp
1 Tbsp	1/4 tsp	6 – 9 drops
1 tsp	pinch – 1/16 tsp	2 – drops

. . . . .

Xylitol: Another Safe Sweetener

. . . . .

Another good and sweet health benefit is low-cal Xylitol according to C.J. Puotinen. In *Good and Sweet Health Benefit*, he tells us that the average American consumes half a cup of sugar every day and that is a lot if you are at risk for diabetes. Xylitol (Pronounced ZY-Ii-tol) can be used if you have insulin resistance, syndrome X, obesity, candida-related yeast infections, tooth decay or other health problems involving too much sweet stuff.

Because Xylitol has the same sweetness as sugar, it can replace sugar in cooking and baking. It dissolves more slowly than sugar at cold temperatures and faster than sugar at warmer temperatures. As unfamiliar as xylitol is to most of us, it is familiar to our bodies. Humans produce about 15 grams of xylitol each day. This helps explain why most people tolerate small doses very well. There are numerous products available to us that are sweetened with xylitol.

It does have some health benefits, we are told, for those who may have recurring sinus problems. Xylitol nasal washes or inserts prevent bacteria from adhering to nasal tissue and mucous membranes of upper respiratory passages, thus preventing infection. The same mechanism helps prevent ear infections. According to John Peldyak, DMD, who has written extensively about xylitol, he says the next breakthroughs in his xylitol research are likely to occur in body building and sports nutrition, because xylitol is efficiently and steadily converted to glucose (energy) and glycogen (storage). It may be particularly useful when coupled with other carbohydrates for recovery after heavy exercise.

Xylitol has been tested extensively for safety. In 1963, the US Food and Drug Administration (FDA) approved xylitol as a dietary supplement and nutritional sweetener. The only side effect reported in humans is that if used in large amounts it may produce intestinal gas and diarrhea. They say there are no well-known drug interactions with xylitol.

CHAPTER EIGHT

CHOLESTEROL AND TRANS FATS

W HEN I WENT AWAY TO SCHOOL, I loved the yucky white bread and all the luscious pastries. My diet as I had grown up with changed completely and eventually my health began to fail.

My husband Phil did extensive research and taught in his classes that prevention is the key to fighting illnesses such as heart disease and cancer. Cholesterol build-up in the arteries increases the risk of heart disease.

We have a problem with cholesterol, which is a fatty wax-like substance made by the liver. It is necessary for the production of hormones, Vitamin D, and bile. Our bodies produce all the cholesterol we need. So, we should know what foods contain cholesterol.

There is good and bad cholesterol. The good

carries the "bad "cholesterol to the liver to be broken down and removed from the body; the "bad" cholesterol or LDL carries the cholesterol from the liver through the bloodstream causing a build-up in the blood vessels. To avoid this, we must limit our intake of high-cholesterol foods and unhealthy fats. Good food choices would be foods high in fiber such as beans, peas, oatmeal, barley, grains, brown rice, apples, oranges, carrots, dried fruit, oats and wheat brans.

We are reminded that sweets, white sugar, white flour, and fatty foods may lead to a health problem. Most doctors recommend limiting these types of foods, as they do nothing to build but tend to cause the body to become acidic. Then illnesses can take over. It is recommended that we eat more fruits, vegetables and whole grains, which contain sterols to help block the absorption of cholesterol. So many people never make a connection between what they put in their mouths and their general health. Many people grow up eating junk foods and things that taste good but are not nutritious.

We will explore other cholesterol awareness and cautions in the section to come on Trans Fat and Saturated Fat Concerns.

If only we could know and be taught how detrimental some foods and drinks are to our health. We should be taught that it is not good to eat excessive amounts of red meat with all the hormones, pork which is very acidic, processed foods, soda drinks, homogenized milk from hormone-fed cows (get the book at the library *Milk A to Z*), monster drinks and soda pop, which are bad for our health as well as too many carbohydrates such as starches and sugars.

Wrong combinations of foods are harmful to our bodies too. Certain foods require particular digestive enzymes and factors for proper digestion. It can be confusing to our digestive system to be unaware of the combinations our bodies require. We should think about food and enzyme combinations so foods can be digested properly.

Proteins and vegetables go well together. Fruits digest rather quickly so they should be eaten alone. Starches such as potatoes, bread, pasta, etc., are best not eaten with meats and proteins. When God created Adam and Eve, they ate from the garden i.e. fruit in season, vegetables in season, meat eaten sparingly. Mostly in the winter when other foods were not plentiful, they ate meat to keep warm.

Our bodies would digest our foods better if we ate accordingly and they would not be confused and weakened. Our pancreas must work extra hard to do its job when we eat starches and protein foods at the same time. Digestion starts in the mouth, so we should thoroughly chew our food at least 23 times before it goes to the pancreas.

Live foods contain enzymes that combine with saliva as we chew, which makes it easier for the pancreas to do its job. When food is cooked over 105°, enzymes are destroyed. Thus it is important to eat at least 80 percent live and 20 percent cooked foods to ensure good health.

So many of us grow up eating a breakfast of perhaps a slice of white-bread toasted, slathered with butter or margarine, and with lots of jam made with white sugar; a bowl of processed cereal with homogenized milk; and gulping down a vitamin pill before running off to school or work—but we are not nutritionally fed. Our bodies are building new cells constantly and what we put into our mouths determines whether or not we are building strong healthy nourished cells or unhealthy cells. If the food is not nutritious we build unhealthy cells on top of unhealthy cells. This leads to illnesses. If we feed our bodies properly then we build strong healthy cells and stay well. It is so simple.

This type of diet would help the body to rebuild in so many ways. Some foods are animal products such as beef, chicken, eggs, and dairy products and should be eaten sparingly. High cholesterol causes hardening of the arteries, narrowing and clogging the blood vessels. This in turn decreases oxygen flow to the heart and can cause heart attacks and stroke, which of course may cause disabilities or even death.

Men 45 years and older, women 55 years and older should have their cholesterol checked regularly because the same things that cause heart disease mentioned above also cause excess cholesterol. I had high cholesterol and when my doctor wanted to put me on a cholesterol lowering statin drug, I asked him if I could try something first that had been suggested by a friend, which was Red Yeast Rice. He agreed. When I went back to him he was amazed that it had brought my cholesterol down and wanted to know more about it.

Sherry A. Rogers, M.D. wrote an article on "Know Your Cholesterol: Myths and Tips," the real deal on statins, natural remedies and more. She wrote: "You have been told that you have high-cholesterol and need to take cholesterol-lowering medication for the rest of your life. If you don't, cholesterol will glue itself to the lining of your heart blood vessels and you'll die of a sudden heart attack or stroke. (My cardiologist told this to me eight years ago). But Dr. Rogers stated that this is wrong. Cholesterol by itself is not the villain. Furthermore, controlling your cholesterol doesn't guarantee that you won't have a heart attack.

Phil also mentioned that a diet for low cholesterol is difficult, as we know the liver make 80 percent of our cholesterol regardless of diet.

We know our bodies need sufficient cholesterol and the right fats to stay healthy. If our cholesterol is high, it's important that we should stick to a healthy whole-foods diet. We can enjoy grains such as quinoa, which I soak and sprout for use in salads, with fruits or vegetables to make them even more nutritious.

And did you know that half of the individuals who have had heart attacks don't have high cholesterol? Cracking some common myths about cholesterol and ditching the class of cholesterol-lowering drugs known as statins for nonprescription, inexpensive nutrients can help you get back on the path toward better health. What you learn about cholesterol may surprise you.

A healthy body needs cholesterol. It is essential to prevent Alzheimer's disease and is crucial for building hormones, making bile for digestion and detoxification, and much more. In fact, cholesterol that's too low is dangerous. Low cholesterol dramatically damages mental health, leading to depression, mania and other problems. It can cause irregular heartbeat, chest pain, high blood pressure and shortness of breath.

Another myth is that statin drugs are the answer for lowering cholesterol. She writes that for anyone taking these drugs (Lipitor, Mevacor, Zocor, and

Crestor to name a few) these drugs can usher in dangerous side effects and seemingly unrelated diseases. Symptoms and side effects of statins include bloating, diarrhea, and constipation, which invariably lead to intestinal inflammation and poor absorption of nutrients—which in turn may lead to an avalanche of diseases. The TV ads for some of those statin drugs actually list decline and death as possible side effects, while beautiful music plays and people are involved in happy activities to distract us from the disturbing disclaimers.

Dr. Rogers also stated that the statin drugs work by poisoning a liver enzyme that makes cholesterol. We need cholesterol to keep the brain from aging.

Statin drugs turn off cholesterol production, which fuels the Viagra epidemic, because you need cholesterol to make sex hormones like testosterone, estrogen, and progesterone.

We need cholesterol to properly release the chemicals we make inside our cells to kill cancer cells and if these side effects weren't enough, the same enzyme that statins inhibit is used by the body to make coenzyme CoQ10. This vitamin-like substance is necessary and statin drugs actually create a life-threatening deficiency in CoQ10.

People taking statin drugs eventually develop a host of diseases caused by a deficiency of this nutrient including congestive heart failure and heart attacks, exhaustion, cancer, muscle disease, depression, high blood pressure, gum disease, hair loss, liver disease, memory loss, cataracts, folic acid deficiency and much more.

Reading Dr. Roger's writings I have thought If we know our choices and understand our bodies, doesn't it seem prudent that we should at least try to help ourselves instead of taking our bodies in to our overworked doctors saying 'fix my body, as we take our car into the garage, and asked them to fix it.'

She did note in her article that if you are on statin drugs; start taking CoQ10 as soon as possible. (Costco has sales often on the liquid form). Vitamin E that contains all eight parts. Taking four tocopherois and four tocotrienols has also been helpful along with CoQ10. It is important to avoid synthetic di-tocopherol and always choose the natural d-alpha-tocopherol.

She added a tip: there are safer, cheaper, and better alternatives to improve cholesterol. Vitamin B3, or niacin is a wonderful nature's way to lower cholesterol and is one of the oldest, safest, and best-researched. Niacin not only safely decreases cholesterol synthesis but also raises HDL and helps lower triglycerides. Look for a formula that allows slow release over five to seven hours.

Keep it up until you find the cause and cure for your high cholesterol and you and your doctor can eliminate the statin. I mentioned before that Red Yeast Rice does seem to help.

My dear Doctor B suggested that I take niacin when I refused to take the drugs. He had said before that he wouldn't treat me if I didn't do as he suggested. Then he said he didn't mean that, as I had the pacemaker and he had to check it periodically. I don't think he knew quite what to do with me but now he tells me I am doing great. I will always be grateful for him as he found out what my heart problem was after suffering and not knowing what my problem was or getting answers from my previous doctors for a very long time.

It was mentioned also that a diet for low cholesterol is difficult to achieve, as we know the liver makes 80 percent of our cholesterol regardless of our diet. And our bodies need sufficient cholesterol and the right fats to stay healthy. If our cholesterol is high, we should just stick to a healthy whole-foods diet. Enjoy grains such as brown rice and quinoa.

Dr. Rogers says Vitamin C is needed to finish converting cholesterol into bile, necessary for absorbing fat-soluble nutrients the likes of Vitamins A, D, E, and K plus CoQ10, and other nutrients necessary for a normal cholesterol level.

Magnesium, the Nutrient
Most Diets Are Deficient In

As many as 8 out of 10 Americans may be lacking magnesium, the nutrient that's essential for memory and general brain health, detoxification, energy metabolism, glutathione production and the optimization of your mitochondria. In short, magnesium has enormous potential to influence your health and general well-being, especially the prevention of heart disease and cancer, but also for general energy and athletic performance.

Because there's no reliable way to assess your body's levels, sometimes the only clue you get that you're low is when the following red flags appear, as reported by Dr. Mercola:

Magnesium is the fourth most abundant mineral in your body and is involved in more than 600 different biochemical reactions. Research suggests even subclinical deficiency can jeopardize your heart health.

A lack of magnesium will impede your cellular metabolic function and deteriorate mitochondrial function. Magnesium deficiency has been identified as the greatest predictor of heart disease. This nutrient is required both for increasing the number of mitochondria in your cells and for increasing mitochondrial efficiency.

Magnesium is also important for chromosome folding,

which allows cells to divide, multiply and regenerate to make up for lost or damaged cells. Check your RBC magnesium level and track signs and symptoms of magnesium insufficiency to determine how much magnesium you need.

Low potassium and calcium are also common laboratory signs indicating magnesium deficiency. To optimize your magnesium level, eat magnesium-rich foods and/or take a magnesium supplement.

Taking Epsom salt baths is another effective way to boost your magnesium level.

Magnesium assists in the metabolism of calcium, potassium, zinc, phosphorous, iron, sodium, hydrochloric acid, acetylcholine and nitric oxide, as well as 300 enzymes and the activation of thiamine.

Magnesium is also required for DNA, RNA and protein synthesis and integrity, and plays a role in the creation of chromosomes.

Regulation of blood sugar and insulin sensitivity, which is important for the prevention of Type 2 diabetes. In one study, 10 pre-diabetics with the highest magnesium intake reduced their risk for blood sugar and metabolic problems by 71 percent. Relaxation of blood vessels and normalizing blood pressure are assisted by magnesium.

Muscle and nerve function, including the action of your heart muscle, are enhanced with essential magnesium.

Magnesium is a catalyst in mood regulation, working like serotonin to prevent anxiety and depression as an *important stress antidote. Other brain support includes preventing migraine headaches.*

It is an important nutrient for helping to maintain normal blood pressure and protect against stroke. Author Dr. Andrea Rosanoff, Ph.D., reported, "Numerous studies found low magnesium associated with all known cardiovascular risk factors, such as cholesterol, high blood pressure, hardening of the arteries and the calcification of soft tissues."

As explained by British cardiologist Dr. Sanjay Gupta, a prescribed number of magnesium capsules support heart health via a variety of different mechanisms. For starters, it combats inflammation, thereby helping prevent hardening of your arteries and high blood pressure. It also improves blood flow by relaxing your arteries, and helps prevent your blood from thickening, allowing it to flow more smoothly. All of these basic effects are important for optimal heart function.

Most people need an additional 300 mg of magnesium per day in order to lower their risk of developing numerous chronic diseases.

In a 2016 meta-analysis, 20 of 40 studies involving more than 1 million participants in nine countries found that, compared to those with the lowest magnesium intakes, those with the highest magnesium intakes had:

- 10 percent lower risk of coronary heart disease
- 12 percent lower risk of stroke
- 26 percent lower risk of Type 2 diabetes

Increasing magnesium intake by 100 mg per day lowered participants' risk for:

- Heart failure by 22 percent
- Stroke by 7 percent
- Diabetes by 19 percent
- All-cause mortality by 10 percent

It is sad that more people won't take control of their lives. Many of us seem to eat and overeat without thinking of nutrient value. People who are deficient in magnesium are most likely to have a sudden cardiac arrest. This mineral prevents blood clots, dilates blood vessels, and can also stop the development of dangerous heart irregularities. It is equally important for bones and body tissue.

Beyond supplements, what foods contain magnesium in sufficient quantities to be of use to our bodies?

Nuts are rich in magnesium. Pecans, for example, are very high in magnesium as are seeds. Pumpkin seeds especially, rich dark chocolate, green leafy vegetables, whole grains, bananas, avocados and fish are all excellent sources of magnesium.

. . . . .

Grow Your Own Nutrient-Rich Foods

. . . . .

It is so good to maintain a little garden spot, or as I do, fill several big pots with organic soil on the patio and grow lettuce, spinach, parsley, green onions, beets and carrots. Swiss chard and kale will withstand the cold weather, as will some other vegetables. I pick the leaves off for salads and let the plants keep growing all season.

Kale is a leafy vegetable that grows the year round in my area, and is so great to put in your healthy, easy-to-make smoothie drinks. Spinach and lettuce do not like the heat. I plant them in the summer and by the time they are coming up the weather is cooling down. I enjoy fresh veggies all winter long.

In St. George, Utah, where people come to spend the winters, the weather is. mild. I plant peas in November and have peas early in the spring. I love to eat them—as well as asparagus—raw.

Vitamin D, which is found in sunshine, fish, orange juice, and is added to pasteurized cows' milk—which we never drink—but for those who do, Vitamin D is so important to our bodies. Most women do not get enough Vitamin D, especially in winter months. Lack of Vitamin D3 can result in heart failure, heart attack, stroke, and it puts us at a definite risk for adverse cardiovascular problems. Vitamin D also helps fight the flu.

. . . . .

AN AMINO ACID, L-ARGININE IS ANOTHER ESSENTIAL NUTRIENT

. . . . .

Amino acids function in building, growth and repair of our body's cells. They may also act as free-radical scavengers and neurotransmitters.

L-arginine, an amino acid is very important for our bodies. It is converted in the body into a chemical called nitric oxide, which is a chemical building block used for heart and blood vessel conditions including congestive heart failure, chest pain, high blood pressure and coronary artery disease. It is used with chemotherapy drugs for treatment of breast cancer.

We could list more than 20 other amino acid types, but you can research them on line or at your natural food stores and holistic experts.

Some people use L-arginine for preventing the common cold, improving kidney function after a kidney transplant, combating high blood pressure, improving athletic performance, boosting the immune system and preventing inflammation of the digestive tract in premature infants.

L-arginine is used in combination with many over-the-counter and prescription medications for a variety of conditions. For example, it is used along with ibuprofen for migraine headaches, and with fish oil and other supplements for reducing infections, improving wound healing and shortening recovery time following surgery.

. . . . .

Trans Fat and Saturated Fat Concerns

. . . . .

Dr. Suzanne Havala Hobbs, Ph.D. from the University of North Carolina at Chapel Hill reports it has been some time since the FDA began requiring that the trans-fat content of processed foods be listed on the nutrition-fact labels. She adds that since this regulation went into effect, many food manufacturers have stopped using this harmful type of fat. However, not all foods are free of trans fats. And it may be 'hidden' unless you know what to look for on food labels. She explains how trans-fat is bad for our health. It raises LDL, the 'bad' cholesterol, and lowers 'good' HDL cholesterol and increases inflammation in the body, which is a risk factor for heart disease, diabetes, cancer and other serious medical conditions.

Trans fat has been used since the early 1900s when food scientists discovered that if they pumped hydrogen through liquid vegetable oil, it turned into a viscous substance, known as partially hydrogenated oil. The substance makes food flakier when cooked and extends the shelf life of food in the grocery stores. It became a mainstay in margarine, commercial baked goods, pastries, cookies, crackers and deep-fried foods as well as frozen dinners, chips and even some cereals.

According to the FDA's trans-fat labeling regulation, a food product can be made to appear to be free of trans fat even if it contains small amounts of the fat. For example, the nutrition facts label of a food that contains trans fat in an amount less than 0.5 g per serving, may claim 'zero trans fat'. Or it may omit a trans-fat listing but include a footnote that reads "Not a significant source of trans fat."

We must read labels for the ingredients and be aware of the legal deceptions on the labels of our store-bought foods. If "partially hydrogenated oil," "shortening" or "vegetable shortening" appears in the ingredients list, the product contains trans fats. But trans-fat is not listed on the nutrition facts label if the food contains less than .05 g per serving of trans fat. Granted this small amount may at first glance seem insignificant, but that is not the case if you consume multiple daily servings of the food, as is common for many people.

Dr. Hobbs notes that some snack foods, such as granola bars, put "zero trans-fat" per serving while listing partially hydrogenated oil among the ingredients. Example: Quaker Cherry Chocolate Chip Granola Bars state zero grams of trans fat per one-bar (24 g) serving but list partially hydrogenated soybean and/or cottonseed oil in the ingredient list. Aunt Jemima Complete Pancake & Waffle Mix also lists zero grams of trans fat per serving (two four-inch pancakes), yet the ingredient list includes partially hydrogenated soybean oil.

Some products promoted for their health benefits also contain partially hydrogenated oil such as Benecol, a supposedly healthy replacement for butter or margarine.

She warns that we need to be aware that some meats and dairy products contain small amounts of trans fat, in a naturally occurring form. Their saturated fat content is a far more significant health concern. Saturated fat is found in whole milk, cheese, butter, ice cream and red meat. Saturated fat has long been known to increase heart disease risk by raising cholesterol levels.

Dr. Hobbs advised that when evaluating a food product, add the grams of trans fat and saturated fat together. Limit your combined *daily* total intake of these fats to the recommended intake for saturated fat alone (20 g for people consuming 2,000 calories in a day).

She adds that it is important to note the polyunsaturated fat found in corn, soybean and safflower oils, and the mono-unsaturated fat found in olives, avocados, nuts, and olive, canola and peanut oils have the opposite effect. These fats reduce heart disease risk by lowering LDL and raising HDL levels.

Polyunsaturated and monounsaturated fats generally are found in foods of plant origin, and these fats remain liquid at room temperature. Most saturated fats come from animal sources and are solid at room temperature.

Let's now talk about butter and margarine. It was interesting to find out that margarine was originally manufactured to fatten turkeys. When it killed the turkeys, the people who had put all the money into research wanted a payback so they put their heads together to figure out what to do with this product to get their money back. It was a white substance with no food appeal so they added the yellow coloring and sold it to people to use in place of butter. I remember as a child my mother bought it a few times and it was white but had a little oval shaped yellow pill in the plastic package that one would squeeze and massage until it was the color of butter. I remember my Dad having a fit about buying it.

Do we know the difference between margarine and butter? It is interesting that they both have the same number of calories. Butter is slightly higher in saturated fats at 8 grams compared to 5 grams in margarine. Eating margarine can increase heart disease in women by 53 percent over eating the same amount of butter, according to a recent Harvard Medical Study. Margarine is very high in trans fatty acids and triples the risk of coronary heart disease as it increases total cholesterol and bad LDL and lowers good HDL. Margarine increases the risk of cancers up to five-fold. It lowers the quality of breast milk and decreases immune and insulin response.

It is noted that margarine is only one molecule away from being plastic! Can you imagine giving this to your family? If you doubt any of this then do a test by purchasing a tub of margarine and leave it in your garage or shaded area. Within a couple of days, you will note a couple of things: no flies—not even those pesky fruit flies—will go near it (that alone should tell us how worthless it is). It does not rot or smell differently because it has no nutritional value. Nothing will grow on it because it is nearly plastic. We might as well melt Tupperware and spread it on toast!

Eating butter increases the absorption of many other nutrients in other foods but is a saturated fat and isn't as good as it was before they began to use so many hormone shots and chemicals in cattle feed. It does have many nutritional benefits where margarine has a few only because they are added. Butter tastes much better than margarine and it can enhance the flavor of other foods. Butter has been around for centuries but regardless, one has to limit saturated fats if possible.

Some people soften organic butter and add olive oil or flax-seed oil, mixing well to extend the quantity, thus lessoning the amount of saturated fat intake.

CHAPTER NINE

STROKE AND CARDIOVASCULAR ILLNESSES

W E SHOULD ALL BE AWARE of the warning signs of heart attacks and strokes. We are told by the American Heart Association that heart and blood vessel disease is our nation's number one killer. We should know what to do if we suspect a heart attack.

Some warning signs are: chest discomfort, or discomfort in other areas of the upper body, and shortness of breath, with or without chest discomfort. Other signs include nausea, or severe indigestion, pain along the jaw, light-headedness or a cold sweat.

Stroke is the third highest cause of death and if survived, the possible cause of long-term disability. Stroke affects the arteries of the brain. It occurs when a blood vessel bringing blood to the brain gets blocked or ruptures so brain cells don't get the flow of oxygenated blood they need. Deprived of oxygen, nerve cells can't function and die within minutes. The part of the body controlled by these nerves permanently can't function because dead brain cells can't be replaced.

My husband did a lot of research on cayenne pepper and found how it had a tendency to clean out the arteries to the brain. It has been suggested that Phosfood Liquid from Standard Process Labs is something to have on hand in case of a stroke. A dropper full in water taken immediately while medical help is being sought may help to prevent debilitation. Continue to take it every hour until medical help arrives.

Warning signs of a stroke may be: a sudden weakness or numbness of the face, arm or leg, especially on one side of the body. Sudden confusion, trouble speaking or understanding; difficulty seeing in one or both eyes; sudden difficulty in walking; dizziness; loss of balance or coordination; severe headache; sagging of one side of the face; or the inability to lift both arms equally. Don't wait, immediately call 911 or the Emergency Medical Services, (EMS) in your area (fire department or ambulance). Or call a friend or neighbor. It is not wise to drive yourself.

Talk to your doctor, or health-care professionals

to become knowledgeable about stroke symptoms. The American Stroke Association can be reached at 1-888-4-stroke or visit them online at www. StrokeAssociation.org.

To know if you are at risk you can do a peripheral arterial disease (PAD) self-test as follows:

- Do you have cardiovascular (heart) problems such as high blood pressure, heart attack or stroke?

- Do you have diabetes?

- Do you have a family history of any of the above?

- Do you have aching, cramping or pain in your legs when you walk or exercise but then the pain goes away when you rest?

- Do you have pain in your toes or feet at night?

- Do you have any ulcers or sores on your feet or legs that are slow in healing?

- Do you smoke? Or have you in the past?

- Are you more than 25 pounds overweight?

- Do you eat fried or fatty foods three times a week or more?

- Do you have an inactive lifestyle?

The more yes answers you have to those questions, the more important it is to change your diet and lifestyle and see your doctor.

All this information is from the American Heart Association.

We should understand and know the causes and effects of stroke and cardiovascular illnesses before we can begin to help ourselves.

. . . . .

HIGH BLOOD PRESSURE EXPLAINED

. . . . .

What is high blood pressure and what causes it? Blood pressure is the force of the blood pushing against the walls of the arteries. The causes of high blood pressure vary but may include narrowing of the arteries causing the heart to work harder than it should. Nearly one in three American adults have high blood pressure, as reported by the American Heart Association.

Many Americans tend to develop this condition as they get older but it is not part of healthy aging. We can help ourselves if we know the risk factors such as family history, aging, lifestyle and race. African Americans are more likely to develop high blood pressure than Caucasians. People with diabetes are at a greater risk as well.

Before having your blood pressure taken, for a better result avoid eating or drinking anything other than water 30 minutes before the test, empty your bladder and wait for at least five minutes with your feet flat on the floor. Have two or more readings and average the results. Keep a record of your blood-pressure readings.

Phil saved an article from our local newspaper back in 2010 in the "Health Life" column written by Kristy Ann Pike. "Prevention Is Key" when it comes to heart health. She reported that statistics show most of us will deal with cardiovascular disease sooner or later as it is the number one killer for U. S. adults every year. She also wrote that Dr. Jamison Jones of Heart of Dixie Cardiology said some patients came to him hoping for a "silver bullet" that would take care of their heart problem.

He suggested that apparently exercise and prevention are really the keys to avoiding cardiovascular diseases, according to the American Heart Association and the American College of Cardiology.

We should exercise at least 30 minutes daily; the more you work your body the greater the benefit to your health. A brisk walk five times a week is good. How blessed are those who live in an area where there is abundant clean air, sunshine and beautiful scenery.

WOMEN AND HEART DISEASE

There are things every woman should know about heart disease. We tend to ignore some of the signs. If our husbands have a chest pain we immediately call 911 but our symptoms are sometimes deceptive and we don't realize what is happening.

Symptoms can be shortness of breath, jaw or back pain, nausea, light-headedness or feeling dizzy. We may take something thinking it will go away and therefore more women do not survive heart attacks.

Women are especially susceptible if they take or have taken birth control pills, if they smoke or if they are having hormone treatments. Hormones prescribed to ease the symptoms of menopause may increase risk also.

Women must protect themselves by not being overweight and learning how to manage stress.

Some ways we can help to control our blood pressure are to be physically active, maintain a healthy weight, limit alcohol, quit smoking, try a dietary approach, choose foods with low sodium, decrease saturated fats, eat less red meat, dairy, breads made with white flour, and limit or avoid sweets.

Consume more whole grains, nuts, walnuts, pecans, almonds, seeds such as sunflower, flax, sesame, chia seeds and remember to soak all seeds and nuts overnight in purified water to release the enzyme inhibitor that keeps them from growing so they will reproduce the next generation the following year. This inhibitor is hard for us to digest so by soaking, draining and letting nuts and seeds sprout they are so much easier to digest and more nutritious for us.

If you prefer them crisp, one can soak, drain and sprout (rinsing often) and then dehydrate. I even soak dried beans overnight, drain, put in a colander, cover with damp towel to keep them moist and dark until a little sprout appears, rinsing them often, prior to cooking them. I do this with brown rice also. The food value increases. It takes less cooking time also after being sprouted and they even have a better flavor.

Eat more fruits and vegetables such as sweet potatoes, avocados, zucchinis, beets, celery, carrots. Cabbage, etc., garlic seems to help decrease high blood pressure and of course cayenne pepper to help the arteries. Eat live foods when possible.

Google live-food recipes—there are so many available. NOTE: *Chapter 16* in this book offers recipes for achieving optimum health.

Avoid canned or processed foods as much as

possible. If you must use them drain and rinse
to remove some of the salt. I make a mixed bean
salad with whole corn and canned beans, which my
husband loved.

CHAPTER TEN

THE SECRET OF ENZYMES

L ET'S THINK ABOUT ENZYMES. What are they? They are complex-protein substances produced within plants or animals and will not work without the help of other substances known as co-enzymes. Vitamins and minerals act as co-enzymes and must be obtained from food. Enzymes are biochemical spark plugs for every function of our bodies.

LIPASE—An enzyme that digests fat

PROTEASE—An enzyme that digests protein

AMYLASE—An enzyme that digests carbohy-drates, usually found in the mouth's saliva

Certain enzymes are lipo-proteins composed of essential fats and fatty acids combined with varying amounts and proportions of amino acids. So far as science has been able to discover, the main function of vitamins have is the role they play in supporting enzymes. Every thought, action and reaction the human body is capable of is the result of enzyme activity.

The purpose of enzymes is to destroy toxins, free radicals and antigens in the liver and bloodstream. They enable vitamins, minerals, and amino acids we consume to be converted to vital neurotransmitters—allowing us to see, hear, think, create, and just plain feel good. They are the biological helpers that kick-start all the processes of life. Without them, we would cease to function.

The body manufactures enzymes from nutrients in food. The primary sources of enzymes are raw unpolluted foods. Cooking destroys enzymes so if you must eat mostly cooked foods then be sure to get some good enzymes to take along with your meal. Lipase enzyme digests fat, protease digests protein, and amylase digests carbohydrates usually found in saliva. Thus emphasizing the importance of chewing foods thoroughly, since digestion begins in the mouth—particularly when consuming carbohydrate foods.

All healthy foods in their natural state contain the enzymes required to digest them but because of modern stresses, (including bad food, pesticides, preservatives, hormones, and other additives), our bodies must try to produce far more of the digestive enzymes causing stress. Therefore, as we suggested earlier, soak all seeds and nuts and let them sprout. (Sadly, many seeds and nuts are pasteurized and will not sprout.) Sprouting means these seeds and nuts are pre-digested and full of enzymes. They can be dried after sprouting if one prefers them crispy rather than soft.

For example, heart disease is linked to low levels of the important enzyme CoQ10. A lack of folic acid seems to weaken and destroy arteries. Low levels of vitamin B are linked to Alzheimer disease. People with arthritis always have low levels of pantothenic acid, and people with prostate cancer usually have deficient levels of vitamin E. Many diseases now linked to nutritional deficiencies, are due to our ignorant consumption of unhealthy foods.

In contrast, wheatgrass contains a broad spectrum of vitamins, minerals, antioxidants, amino acids, essential fatty acids and enzymes.

Enzyme supplements as healer elements have been linked to amazing cessations of pain, heart disease and circulatory conditions, skin conditions, cancer, migraines, diabetes, crones disease, autism and eczema.

CHAPTER ELEVEN

THE IMPORTANCE OF pH BALANCE

Alkaline or Acidic

OVER 40 MILLION AMERICANS have kidney and bladder infections, impairment and disease. Incontinence, the new American epidemic, attacks over 29 million American adults. Following a recommended 5-day detox program can help these problems. I am so grateful for Dr. Schulze and the products that he produces that have helped my family and amazingly did for me what neither my doctor nor antibiotics could ever do, which helped to correct my kidney/bladder infection. Contact his retail store in Marina Del Rey, California. Phone 866-305-9233 Customer Service and request a catalog.

It is said that antibiotics not only kill infections, they kill both the "good" and "bad" bacteria throughout the intestinal tract and leave destruction in their wake.

So many people are sick and have no clue that they can help themselves by taking advantage of the information that is available. If only we will search to find answers and try to help ourselves we can achieve and maintain optimum health. Someone said we are tired of feeling sick and tired and sick and tired of feeling sick and tired and that was how I had felt—that endless unhealthy cycle.

Do you realize that it is a fact that it's medical bills that cause over half of all bankruptcies of American families? Getting healthy and taking responsibility for our own health is really a no-brainer. If we do the things to keep our bodies healthy we can avoid the pain of ill health and the financial stress. Dr. Schulze also has a product called Super Food Plus. Phil had used this for years along with cayenne pepper and he was quite healthy. He outlived all his siblings. Super Food Plus will assimilate into your bloodstream and go to work in ten minutes or less. Everything starts with great nutrition and this product is balanced. This product is complete balanced nutrition for our bodies all made by nature.

Commercial vitamin and mineral pills have failed in many cases. People buy bottles of different vitamins, often spending a fortune on them, which can cause an imbalance doing harm to their bodies.

Dr. Bruce West stated that real healing can only

come from real nutrition. Many of the supplements people are taking are simply chemical ingredients and can even be toxic.

The next time you feel like having a soda, think about how acidic it is. Colas are very acidic with a pH of approximately 2.5. It takes 32 glasses of water with a pH of 1– to neutralize that one cola. It is good that we can be an example for our children and let them know how it is so important to think about what we are putting into our bodies.

We would be wise to maintain an intake ratio of 80 percent alkaline foods and 20 percent acid foods. All fruits and vegetables are alkaline. That includes citrus fruits which are acid until they combine with our saliva and become alkaline. Many foods we can enjoy are alkaline. Among them are: oats, millet, rye, flax, almonds, Brazil nuts, coconut, and lima beans.

When your body is predominantly acid, disease results. Research has found almost all diseases are linked to acid-based yeast and fungus dominance. Watch for the following signs of severe pH imbalance:

- Fatigue/low energy
- Irritability/Mood swings
- Unexplained aches and pains
- Indigestion

- Overweight conditions
- Colitis/Ulcers
- Low resistance to illness
- Diarrhea/Constipation
- Allergies
- Urinary tract infections
- Unbalanced blood sugar
- Rectal/vaginal itch
- Headache

If the alkaline-acid ratio drops to 3 to 1, health is seriously menaced. Should that ratio drop to 2-1/2 to 1, death is imminent. Life is possible only in the presence of an adequate and positive alkaline condition of the body tissues and blood, according to Arthur W. Snyder, Ph.D. researcher.

Try to get your children to eat alkaline foods such as sprouts, one of the most alkalizing foods. My little great grandson used to sit in his high chair—while I was doing all my cancer program then—and I would put different sprouted-seed grains such as sunflower, alfalfa, broccoli, etc. on his tray and he loved them. He is twenty-four now and still loves healthy foods. Sprouted seeds and nuts have an abundance of enzymes and they contain a greater concentration of vitamins, minerals, proteins, phytochemicals, anti-oxidants, nitrosamines, trace minerals, bioflavonoids and chemo-protectants (such as suphoraphane and isoflavone).

. . . . .

How to Test Your pH Balance

. . . . .

First thing when you wake, before drinking, eating or brushing your teeth, work up saliva in your mouth two times and swallow each time. The third time, keep a little saliva on your tongue. Tear off 1/3 of one pH strip and place it on your tongue for 5 seconds. Remove quickly and set it down on a clean dry surface. DO NOT HOLD THE pH STRIP IN YOUR FINGERS. Doing that will change the reading.

The color of the strip will be a shade of gray, white, yellow, green, blue or black. The ideal color is blue (7.0–7.5) if you are neutral and healthy—a good pH balance.

Colors of yellow or green (5.5–6.8) indicate an acidic condition that is unhealthy. Gray and white (3.0–4.5) are very acidic, very unhealthy. The color black indicates extreme acidosis (7.7–14.0) of a diseased body. The kidneys produce ammonia to help raise the pH to neutral.

When the pH strip dries it will return to the

goldfish color of the untested strip.

Acidic foods are: any kind of meat, eggs, milk products (with the exception of whole raw milk), grains, breads, cereals, pastas, anything made with flour, corn products, peanuts, lentils and walnuts.

. . . . .

Signs Your Body Is Too Acidic

. . . . .

I have heard friends say I just can't get my children to enjoy eating healthy things. And it is how they are raised as part of their diet from the time they are tiny. If they are fed lots of sugary sweets and processed foods then their taste buds will reject good healthy food. Mothers living on a tight budget should learn to sprout seeds and serve them to their children to keep them healthy. Sprouts are especially important in the wintertime when fresh vegetables in the stores are declining and becoming more expensive. One can add sprouts to salads, eat them raw or add them to meatloaves, casseroles, soups, stews and juices to increase their nutritional value. Replace lettuce for sprouts like alfalfa and sunflower on sandwiches and tacos. Sprouts are delicious on peanut or almond butter sandwiches! Sprinkle them on top of soups and salads.

Dr. Robert Young indicated that we will have

a 96 percent reduction for insulin needs if we alkalize our diets. All foods and liquids have a pH value that can be measured. Our bodies are made up of seventy 70 percent fluids. To maintain optimum health these fluids should be 7.36 pH. The measurement of urine and/or saliva to determine the body's pH level for acidity has become popular in the alternative medical field. When the body's buffering system is malfunctioning or overloaded, the blood and body fluids in which cells rest become too acidic. We know that most enzymes and other cellular components operate best within a narrow range of pH, the level is usually slightly alkaline.

Likewise, many dormant (latent) viruses in the body are activated when acidity is too high (a low pH). For example, people often notice they get mouth ulcers when they eat too many acidic foods such as pineapple, ketchup or tomatoes. The minerals in the bones serve as one of the body's main buffering systems.

When the blood is too acidic, more calcium is released from the bones to buffer the acidity. This can lead to osteoporosis to a severe calcium-loss degree, promoting fractures and other problems.

The best buffering system is a diet high in vegetables. They contain high levels of magnesium and potassium and those two elements have been shown to best prevent osteoporosis because they are powerful acid buffers.

Our pH levels depend upon what we put into out mouths. Think of it as our "Energy Bank" as we deposit and withdraw money from the bank. The foods we eat withdraw (acid) or deposit (alkaline) energy. *Alkalize or Die* is an informative book written by Dr. Theodore A. Baroody.

It is important that we keep our bodies' pH balanced, not too alkaline, nor too acidic. Drinking 2 ounces of wheatgrass juice daily and a proper diet will help our bodies to stay healthy.

There is a company called InnerLight, which carries a product called SuperGreens. This apparently is a powerful blend of organic grasses, vegetables, sprouted grains, leaves and high-frequency minerals which alkalize, energize and nourish cells as they balance the body's pH level, especially if wheatgrass juice is not available. These all-natural plant ingredients help neutralize acid and pull the blood and tissue balance back to its ideal, more alkaline state.

Liquid Chlorophyll is identical to our hemoglobin except for the center atom (magnesium as opposed to iron). Research indicates as we increase our consumption of chlorophyll the quality and quantity of the red blood cells improve. SuperGreens can apparently be added to water to improve the concentration of this powerful blood builder.

One can find lists of alkaline foods on the Internet. These lists include most vegetables, which are alkaline. Also: lemons, seasonal fruit, salmon, trout, free- range turkey, distilled water and reverse osmosis, almond milk, rice, quinoa, spelt, nuts and seeds (raw and unsalted) Make up a shopping list and keep these in your refrigerator.

A diet made of 80 percent fresh raw vegetables, whole grains, seeds, nuts and a little fruit help put the body into an alkaline environment. After you know you are on the road to recovery you may have perhaps 20 percent cooked foods. We know cancer cells thrive in an acidic environment, so maintaining an alkaline pH is vital.

A meat-based diet is acidic and it is best to only eat a small amount of fish or if you must have meat, only a small amount of range-fed, no hormone, organic chicken or turkey. Other meats contain livestock antibiotics, growth hormones and parasites, which are all harmful, especially to people with cancer. Be aware that meat protein is difficult to digest and requires a lot of digestive enzymes. Undigested meat remains in the intestines and becomes putrefied, leading to more toxic buildup.

Herman Aihara, in his book *Acid & Alkaline*, states that if the condition of our extra cellular fluids, especially the blood, becomes acidic, our physical condition will first manifest tiredness, be prone to catching colds, etc. When these fluids become more acidic, our condition then manifests pains and suffering such as headaches, chest pains, stomach aches, etc. Back in the '90s when I was sick all the time and had all these symptoms, I went to my chiropractor. I would go to his office every morning and he would check my acid/alkaline levels. He is the one that told me to go to an oncologist, as he was so sure that it was cancer because my body was so acidic.

We can check our own levels by purchasing the tape at the health food store and checking our saliva or urine daily before drinking water or eating food to be sure we are keeping an alkaline pH balance in our bodies.

According to Keiichi Morishita in his *Hidden Truth of Cancer*, if the blood develops a more acidic condition, then our body inevitably deposits these excess acidic substances in some area of the body, such that the blood will not be able to maintain an alkaline condition, which causes these areas to become acidic and lowers oxygen.

As this tendency continues, such areas increase in acidity and some cells die: then these dead cells themselves turn into acids. However, some other cells may adapt in that environment. In other words, instead of dying—as normal cells do in an acid environment—some cells survive by becoming abnormal cells. These abnormal cells are called malignant cells and these grow indefinitely and without order and this is CANCER!

[122]

CHAPTER TWELVE

PHARMACEUTICAL DRUGS AND HERBAL ALTERNATIVES

P HIL TAUGHT IN HIS CLASSES that an ounce of prevention involving health matters is still better than a pound of cure—a 16 to 1 ratio. The instruction or prevention information given to us many decades ago is more true and applicable today than it was when it was first given.

Having good health is better than money in the bank. With good health, our potential for earnings is usually assured. Many have learned, through sad experience, that trying to buy one's health back by using prescription drugs, which can be expensive, frustrating, time-consuming and often cause miserable side effects—can be a mistake.

It is noted in our local paper that Utah Legislator Lowry Snow stated that the number four cause of death in the United States is the result of drug poisoning. Since that time the numbers of drug overdoses leading to death have reached epidemic proportions. We are experiencing a national crisis. He said more of our citizens die from unintended prescription opioid drug overdoses than from motor vehicle accidents.

Opioid drugs include those referred to as 'painkillers' and are regularly prescribed by our doctors and dentists to manage pain due to an injury or after a surgical or dental procedure. These pharmaceutical concoctions are extremely addicting and can be lethal even when used as prescribed—or over-prescribed in many cases.

I have a dear friend whose lovely granddaughter injured her shoulder in her work and was prescribed something for pain. Her whole life has been ruined from the addiction.

Legislator Snow warned we should dispose any unused portion properly following the guidelines at www.useonlyasdirected.org or to a permanent collection site or drop-off event. Never take higher doses than prescribed and never share your prescription pain medications with anyone.

Whenever I am diagnosed with a certain ailment I always research it to find the problem and if there are any alternatives to drugs that can be used to overcome it. I know this is frustrating for my doctor but I have always been a determined person and have lived through diphtheria, pneumonia, measles, mumps, chickenpox, polio, cancer and four heart attacks. I have truly been blessed to have survived all of these with the help of my Lord, physicians, my dear husband and also trying to help myself.

Phil's extensive work through the years with research and development testing large liquid propellant rocket engines, using conventional and exotic propellants brought him in daily contact with liquid fluorine, Nitrogen Tetroxide (NT0). Unsymmetrical Dimethyl Hydrazine (UDMH), 95 percent concentrated Hydrogen Peroxide and other chemicals and heavy-metal type propellants clinical tests conducted on him measured concentration of heavy metals. He and his colleagues were regularly tested for levels of these dangerous materials.

When Phil tested positive for heavy metals, he consulted holistic sources for how to rid his body of these pollutants.

. . . . .

Herbal Alternatives to Ridding the Body of Heavy Metal Toxicity

. . . . .

Herbalists suggested we obtain two herbs in dried form: yellow dock root and bugleweed, which are both available at the local health-food stores to help rid Phil's body of heavy metals.

He was instructed to make a tea by using 1 teaspoon of each of the herbs to a cup of boiling water, cover and let steep for 15 minutes. Phil was to drink a cup of this the first thing in the morning and a cup the last thing at night before going to sleep. His instructions were to continue this plan for 30 days and drink lots of pure water also to help flush the toxins from his body.

A clinical laboratory test or iridology test will indicate when your body is rid of the heavy metals. It was further indicted that soaking in a bathtub of hot water containing Epsom Salts will draw toxins from the body to accelerate the cleansing process.

An alternative approach for removing heavy metals from the body can be found in the book *The Cure for All Cancers*, by Dr. Hulda Clark, Ph.D., ND on page 89 of that book.

To remove heavy metals from the body:

1 cup cilantro leaves, packed

6 Tbsp olive oil

Process in a blender of food processor until leaves are minced fine.

Add:

1/2 cup almonds, cashews or walnuts

1 garlic clove

2 Tbsp lemon juice

Blend to the consistency of pesto or dip.
Consume 2 tsp each day for 2 weeks, and repeat annually.
A clay bath is also recommended to remove heavy metals. To the bathtub water, add 1–2 cups of powder or liquid Aztex or Sony clay. Soak for 30 minutes minimum.

————

Dr. Clark reports the use of thioctic acid or lipoic acid capsules, one capsule taken three time per day to trap and prepare for elimination of heavy metals from the body. These are available from Ecological Formulas, Inc. She stated that the statin drugs work by poisoning a liver enzyme that makes cholesterol. However, we need cholesterol to keep the brain from aging. The turn-off cholesterol products fuel the Viagra epidemic, because cholesterol is necessary to create sex hormones like testosterone, estrogen, and progesterone.

We need cholesterol to properly release the chemicals we make inside our cells to kill cancer cells and if these side effects weren't enough, the same enzyme that statins inhibit is used by the body to make coenzyme CoQ10 as stated previously. This vitamin-like substance is necessary and statin drugs create a life-threatening deficiency.

People taking statin drugs eventually develop a host of diseases caused by a deficiency of this nutrient including congestive heart failure and heart attacks, exhaustion, cancer, muscle disease, depression, high blood pressure, gum disease, hair loss, liver disease, memory loss, cataracts, folic acid deficiency and much more.

Reading her text, I have thought, if we know our choices and understand our bodies doesn't it seem prudent that we should at least try to help ourselves instead of taking our bodies in to our overworked doctors saying, "Fix my body, as we take our car into the garage and ask them to fix it."

She did note in her article that if you are on statin drugs, start taking CoQ10 as soon as possible. (Costco has sales often on the liquid). Vitamin E that contains all eight parts, four tocopherols, and four tocotrienols is also helpful. Also, how important to avoid synthetic ditophal and always choose the natural d-alpha-tocopherol.

She added a tip: there are safer, cheaper, and better alternatives to improve cholesterol. Vitamin B3, or niacin is a natural way to lower cholesterol and is one of the oldest, safest, and best researched. Niacin not only safely decreases cholesterol synthesis but also raises HDL and helps lower triglycerides. Look for a formula that allows slow release over five to seven hours.

Continue until you find the cause and cure for your high cholesterol and you and your doctor can eliminate the statin. I mentioned before that Red Yeast Rice does seem to help.

In a Jim Humble newsletter, we were advised to be aware with the following warning:

> *Your government works for the drug companies and the drug companies benefit tremendously if you stay sick all the time, paying money to doctors. That's the way medical system works. No system is evil in itself—only people make it evil. But all you have to do is start thinking for yourself and if you do, you don't have to stay sick or get sick.*

He apparently has taken information from a book *The 24-Hour Diet* by Brian Scott Peskin, B.S.E.E. that he has used successfully in his life time. He claims that there is much misinformation put out by our government in the field of nutrition. Peskin admonishes us not to trust advertising from companies selling foods.

Peskin claims that too much fiber soaks up much-needed nutrients such as vitamins and minerals and is not that healthy. He states that there are no prepared breakfast foods that is really good for our bodies. He asked how could you ever believe that the same people who make money from you—if you are sick—would give you information to make you well and keep you well—free of charge?

You may check him out on Facebook.com/
JimHumbleLive. He claims that something called
MMS and citric acid can be of great value in
preventing many illnesses such as malaria and heart
problems. Phil was very impressed with what he
found when he researched this.

CHAPTER THIRTEEN

CANCER TREATMENTS

D ECADES AGO, European research scientist Dr. Johanna Budwig, who holds a Ph.D. in Natural Science, is one of Germany's premier biochemists and an expert on fats and oils. A six-time Nobel Award nominee, she discovered a totally natural formula. It not only protects against the development of cancer, but fights existing cancer as well. People all over the world who were diagnosed with incurable cancer and sent home to die have greatly benefited from this research and went on to lead normal lives, thanks to this amazing formula.

After 30 years of study, Dr. Budwig observed that the bodies of seriously ill cancer patients were deficient in certain nutrients. It was the lack of these nutrients that allowed cancer cells to grow out of control. By simply eating a combination of two natural and delicious foods—the Budwig flax and organic cottage cheese diet regimen—not only may cancer be prevented, but in case after case it was healed. Other ailments such as strokes, arteriosclerosis, cardiac infarction, fatty degeneration of the liver, poor brain activity, immune deficiency syndromes (MS, autoimmune illnesses) and others were healed as well. It was said because of Dr. Budwig's discovery that symptoms of cancer, liver dysfunction and diabetes could be completely alleviated.

However, when she went to publish these results so that everyone could benefit, drug manufacturers blocked her. They stood to lose a lot of money. Since natural substances cannot be patented, drug companies won't make money by marketing them. To me, this is a crime, and it was my husband's desire that this information be made public so we could all become aware of what is happening. For over 10 years, her methods have proved effective, yet she is denied publication—blocked by the giants who control cancer-"fighting" pharmaceuticals and don't want you to read her words. Do check out her books and read about her.

Dr. Budwig has come up with remarkable natural formulas and diets that work for hundreds and thousands of patients. *How to Fight Cancer and Win* by William L Fischer, who has studied these methods, reveals their secrets to you. You can decide if you want to try them or go for the conventional treatments that may damage your immune system, etc. Pay special attention to page 82 of *How to Fight Cancer and Win* for the delicious diet that can help stop the formation of cancer cells and shrink tumors.

. . . . .

CHEMOTHERAPY

. . . . .

The most common, and most lucrative, treatment for cancer is chemotherapy. But how effective is it really? In the "Cancer Free Newsletter", Dr. Garcia professed that chemotherapy only works about 3 percent of the time! However, most oncologists prescribe and administer this treatment even though many patients suffer far worse side effects than the cancers themselves. Bill Henderson also reports that chemotherapy only works on 12 types of cancer and is only 3 percent effective. However, the Budwig flax oil and organic cottage cheese diet is over 90 percent effective on nearly all types of cancer. Unfortunately, these safe and effective remedies are inexpensive. Phil said it was unfortunate because there's money to be made in pharmaceuticals. Of course, the pharmaceutical companies would rather push deadly poisons because they can make a large profit.

From "Cancer-Free: Your Guide to Gentle, Non-toxic Healing," Dan C. Roehm, M.D. FACP, an oncologist and former cardiologist, wrote an article in 1990 in the *Townsend Letter for Doctors & Patients* saying, "This diet is far and away the most successful anti-cancer diet in the world. What she (Dr. Johanna Budwig) has demonstrated to my initial disbelief but lately, to my complete satisfaction in my practice is cancer is easily curable. The treatment is dietary/lifestyle, the response is immediate; the cancer cell is weak and vulnerable, the precise biochemical breakdown point was identified by her in 1951 and is specifically correctable in vitro (test tube) as well as in vivi (real). Even in difficult cases it is possible to restore health in a few months at most, I would truly say 90 percent of the time. And he states that this has never been contradicted, but this knowledge has been a long time reaching this side of the ocean, hasn't it?

In the *Spotlight Magazine* July 30, 1979, Gale McVay explained her experience with chemotherapy. She said that someone near and dear to her, someone who can never be replaced in her mind and heart, died a premature and totally unnecessary death. This individual had cancer. Although there are safe, effective treatments for this dread disease, methods that do not destroy your body and kill you, as chemotherapy and radiation often do, this person allowed himself to be talked into chemotherapy.

The treatment consisted of some experimental drugs and necessitated a monthly trip at great expense to a large clinic in another state. The side effects of the drugs on this person, her father, were horrendous and unspeakably cruel.

He persevered because he had faith and trust in his doctors, believing every word they told him. He was slowly dying by inches right before their eyes, but he continued taking the awful treatments because his doctors repeatedly told him that he was doing "so well." After all, the good doctors certainly wouldn't lie to him, or would they? She went on to say that the chemo took a tremendous toll on her father and on his loved ones. However, they were powerless to stop the procedures. They took him in for his last treatment, and the prognosis was "very grim". He probably had less than a month to live. Up to that time everything was "rosy" according to his doctors. Her father finally realized he wasn't getting well and agreed to have some non-toxic, humane cancer treatment.

His family took him to the Del Mar Clinic of Dr. Ernesto Contreras in Tijuana, Mexico. There he received metabolic therapy, including Laetrile. With this non-toxic treatment, he was 100 percent more comfortable and relatively free of pain. At least he wasn't hurt or tortured any further and he died a peaceful death. He did not die of cancer, but of pneumonia, one of chemotherapy's most common side effects.

Chemotherapy destroys the body's immune defense system, thereby creating a fertile ground for pneumonia. To a person whose immunity has been destroyed, pneumonia can often be fatal. If her father had understood chemotherapy would not cure him while making his life hell on earth he would never have consented to proceed with it. She goes on to say there is a better way. You do not have to submit to cutting, burning, and poisoning (surgery, radiation, and chemotherapy) for your cancer. She said she vows that her father did not die in vain, and she will continue to do everything to let people know there is an alternative.

Granted most people will take the advice of their doctors and will not investigate any alternative therapies. It is their choice. She remembers the Hippocratic Oath: "First, do not harm. I will prescribe a regimen for the good of my patients according to my ability and judgment and never do harm to anyone. To no one will I prescribe a deadly drug, nor give advice which may cause death." It broke her heart to lose her father, and she prays it doesn't happen to you. I could relate to this dear lady's experience, as this was so much like what happened to our son. But most people will trust their doctors without a doubt, and chemotherapy persists.

Choices We Can Make When Chemotherapy Has Been Prescribed

Southern Utah Life had an article by Kristy Ann Pike where she noted that chances are one out of eight women will suffer from breast cancer and what happens following that diagnosis.

Dr. Derrick Haslem of Dixie Regional Cancer Center in St. George, Utah and Valley View Cancer Center said the treatment recommendations depend upon the woman, her age and overall health, the size of the tumor, how far the cancer has spread and a host of other factors. When the lump is found, mammogram and ultrasound will generally follow to confirm the existence, shape and size of the tumor.

Next, a radiologist performs an ultrasound-guided biopsy, usually under local anesthetic. Tissue obtained will be sent to a lab to check for cancer cells. If it comes back positive, the next stop is the surgeon. If the cancer has spread, it generally goes into the lymph nodes under the armpits, so those areas are checked as well.

After tumor-removal surgery, then consulting with her doctor, "A patient may choose to do nothing," Haslem said.

More often, treatment will consist of a combination of things, including anti-hormone therapy, which is effective in stunting the growth of cancer cells that depend upon estrogen or progesterone to grow.

This is one pill and the prescribed treatment may continue throughout a women's lifetime. Chemotherapy may be mild or aggressive, administered through an IV two-to-four hours at a time, given in between four and eight cycles of two or three weeks each. Radiation usually follows about a month after chemotherapy.

These treatments happen every day, Monday through Friday, for five to six weeks. A machine administers the radiation to a targeted area, generally marked by a tattoo. The entire procedure takes approximately six months. The doctor says after treatment ends, then the most difficult part about having breast cancer is the surveillance period that follows. "Wait and watch" can be more challenging than treatment.

. . . . .

IS CHEMOTHERAPY RIGHT FOR YOU?

. . . . .

Before you go through this torture of your body, do read Dr. Lorraine Day's book and get her opinion. She suggests you find a competent medical professional in your area sympathetic to using alternative, complementary or integrative medicine. Do research. Find out if there is a holistic healer with whom you can connect. Ask people in the medical and health professions, i.e. nurses, doctors, dentists, nutritionists, owners of health food stores, etc. Go to the website and search. Interview each referral and answer the following questions:

- Does the medical professional treat your type of cancer? If the answer is yes, ask if they would be willing to use both alternative and conventional means.

- How do they feel about supplements? If the answer is positive, tell them you hope they can help you, but you are in charge of your own health.

- How long have they been in practice and how much experience do they have with your type of cancer?

- Would they be willing to give the names of three of their patients who would be willing to speak with you?

- Do they accept Medicare?

Keep in mind that some alternative therapists may not be

allowed to treat cancer.

Johns Hopkins' Update had an article stating that after years of telling people chemotherapy is the only way to try *("try" being the key word)* to eliminate cancer, they are finally starting to tell you there is an alternative way. Some of the cancer updates from Johns Hopkins are as follows:

- Every person has cancer cells in their body. These cancer cells do not show up in the standard tests until they have multiplied to a few billion.

When doctors tell cancer patients that there are no more cancer cells in their bodies after treatment, it just means the tests are unable to detect the cancer cells because they have not reached the detectable size or number.

- Cancer cells occur between 6 to more than 10 times in a person's lifetime.
- When the person's immune system is strong, the cancer cells will be destroyed and prevented from multiplying and forming tumors.
- When a person has cancer, it indicates the person has nutritional deficiencies. These could be due to genetic, but also to environmental, food and lifestyle factors.

- Overcome the multiple nutritional deficiencies by changing diet and eating more adequately healthy organic food. Include something like Schulze's Super Food Plus to insure your body is getting the proper amount of nutrients to strengthen your immune systems. Be sure that what you consume is properly balanced so your body can assimilate it. Beware of causing problems of imbalance by selecting foods that are best not consumed in combination or in appropriate quantity. The good Lord gave us natural food to eat so that our bodies could use and build upon them for optimum health.

- Chemotherapy involves poisoning the rapidly growing cancer cells. It also destroys rapidly growing healthy cells in the bone marrow, gastrointestinal tract, etc. and can cause organ damage to liver, kidneys, heart, lungs, etc.

- Radiation, while destroying cancer cells, also burns, scars and damages healthy cells, tissues and organs.

- Initial treatment with chemotherapy and radiation will often reduce tumor size. However prolonged use of both chemo and radiation does not necessarily result in more tumor destruction, we are told.

- When the body has too much toxic burden

from chemo and radiation the immune system is either compromised or destroyed. Hence the person can succumb to various kinds of infections and complications.

· Chemotherapy and radiation can cause cancer cells to mutate and become resistant and difficult to destroy. Surgery can also cause cancer cells to spread to other sites.

· An effective way to battle cancer is to starve the cancer cells by not feeding them with the foods they need to multiply. Sugar, which feeds cancer like squirting gasoline on a fire is a nonfood item to limit severely or avoid altogether. Eliminate all sweets, most sugary fruits, and even carrot juice in the beginning of a cancer-treatment regimen.

·····

ALTERNATIVE METHODS OF TREATING CANCER

·····

BICARBONATE MAPLE SYRUP TREATMENT

The International Medical Veritas Association reported a Bicarbonate Maple Syrup Cancer Treatment, and Bob Livingston posted the following on September 7, 2009: *The bicarbonate maple syrup cancer treatment focuses on delivering natural* chemotherapy in a way that effectively kills cancer cells, but significantly reduces the brutal side effects experienced with most standard chemotherapy treatments. In fact, so great is the reduction that the dangers are brought down to zero. Costs, which are a factor for the majority of people, of this particular treatment are nil.

Though this cancer treatment is very inexpensive, do not assume it is not effective. The bicarbonate maple syrup cancer treatment is a significant cancer treatment every cancer patient should be familiar with, and it can easily be combined with other safe and effective natural treatments.

The actual formula is to mix one-part baking soda from the health food store with three parts maple syrup (pure, 100 percent) in a small saucepan. Stir briskly and heat the mixture for five minutes. Cancer Tutor suggests taking 1 teaspoon daily.

This cancer treatment is similar in principle to Insulin Potentiation Therapy (IPT). IPT treatment consists of giving doses of insulin to a fasting patient sufficient to lower blood sugar into the 50 mg/dl. In a normal person, when you take in sugar, the insulin levels go up to meet the need of getting that sugar into the cells. In IPT they are artificially injecting insulin to deplete the blood of all sugar, then injecting the lower doses of toxic chemo drugs when the blood sugar is driven down to the lowest possible value. It is said that during the low peak the receptors are more sensitive and take on medications more rapidly and in higher amounts. A diabetic friend told me that she was told whenever she eats sweets to eat some protein with it to help keep the insulin levels evenly balanced.

The bicarbonate maple syrup treatment works in reverse to IPT. Roman oncologist Dr. Tullio Simoncini acknowledges that cancer cells gobble up sugar, so when you encourage the intake of sugar it's like sending in a Trojan horse. The sugar is not going to end up encouraging the further growth of the cancer colonies because the baking soda is going to kill the cells before they have a chance to grow.

Instead of artificially manipulating insulin and thus forcefully driving down blood sugar levels to then inject toxic chemo agents, we combine the sugar with the bicarbonate and present it to the cancer cells, which at first are going to love the present. But not for long: This treatment is a combination of pure, 100 percent maple syrup and baking soda and was first reported on the www.CancerTutor.com site. When mixed and heated together, the maple syrup and baking soda bind together. The maple syrup targets cancer cells (which consume 15 times more glucose than normal cells) and the baking soda, which is dragged into the cancer cell by the maple syrup, being very alkaline, forces a rapid shift in pH—thereby killing the cell.

Mark Sircus A.C. also said that perhaps honey could be substituted for maple syrup for those who live in parts of the world where maple syrup is not available, but to his knowledge no one has experimented with this honey ingredient alternative to maple syrup.

"There is not a tumor on God's green earth that cannot be licked with a little baking soda and maple syrup." That is the astonishing claim of controversial folk healer Jim Kelmun who says that this simple home remedy can stop and reverse the deadly growth of cancers. His loyal patients swear by the man they fondly call Dr. Jim and say he is a miracle worker. He also stated that this treatment can be combined with other safe and effective treatments, like transdermal magnesium therapy, iodine, vitamin C, probiotics and other things like plenty of good sun exposure, pure water and clay treatments.

He noted the importance of not using baking soda, which has had aluminum added to it. The Cancer Tutor site reports that the Arm and Hammer brand does have aluminum but the company insists that it is not true. The Bob's Red Mill, Aluminum-free baking soda is safe. He also states that sodium bicarbonate is safe, inexpensive and unstoppably effective when it comes to cancer tissues. It's an irresistible chemical cyanide to cancer cells for it hits the cancer cells with a shock wave of alkalinity, which allows much more oxygen into the cancer cells than they can tolerate. Cancer cells cannot survive in the presence of high levels of oxygen. Studies have already shown how manipulation of tumor pH with sodium bicarbonate enhances some forms of chemotherapy.

It was also noted in this article that Dr. Simoncini suggests the use of sodium bicarbonate, a universal drug like iodine and magnesium chloride. Raising pH increases the immune system's ability to kill bacteria, concludes a study conducted at the Royal Free Hospital and School of Medicine in London. Viruses and bacteria that cause bronchitis and colds thrive in an acidic environment. To fight a respiratory infection and dampen symptoms such as a runny nose and sore throat, taking an alkalizing mixture of sodium bicarbonate and potassium bicarbonate will certainly help. The 1/4 teaspoon each of apple cider vinegar and baking soda taken two times or more a day is another treatment, as is lemon and baking soda, or lime and baking soda formulas.

Vitamin C, l-Lysine and l-Proline Treatment

Dr. Matthias Rath tells us that the next treatment that he would add to the cancer fighting regimen is a mixture of Vitamin C, I-Lysine and I-Proline. The latter two are amino acids. They later added green tea to their formula ingredient list. I read that green tea contains polyphenols and other chemical compounds that reduce inflammation and activate liver enzymes that break down and eliminate potential carcinogens. They found that this combination inhibited the process of metastasis of cancer cells. To find more information on this, go to: http://www4.dr-rath-foundation.org/pdf-files/cancerresearch.pdf.

CLEANLINESS
PREVENTS DISEASE

AS CHILDREN, MANY OF US LEARNED at home that cleanliness is next to Godliness. I've related in the opening chapter about how my mother taught us to wash in the stream outside our modest home before going to bed each night. And there were those weekly baths in the kitchen by the fire. With all of the pollutants in our modern-day environments, keeping our bodies, homes, cars, garages and yards as clean and toxin-free as possible is basic to acquiring and maintaining optimum health.

There are cleaning aids that are alternatives to chemical cleansers. The following examples may prove helpful:

- Ceramic cooking surfaces can be wiped with white vinegar. Let the liquid stand for a few minutes before wiping dry. Be certain to turn off and cool the appliances you are cleaning. Hair spray is effective for stubborn stains.

· To clean an aquarium, if mild soapy water doesn't remove film, spray with hair spray and wipe dry. Rubbing alcohol misted on the glass is also effective.

· To deodorize a musty garage or basement, spread fresh-mown-grass clippings over the floor. Sweep up within a few hours or the next day. The chlorophyll in the grass is a natural deodorizer.

· In place of fabric softener and anti-static-cling products, add a cup of distilled white vinegar to the final rinse. It will deodorize sweaty sports clothing too.

· Hydrogen peroxide is an effective bacteria and virus killer. It is quite preferable to applying antibiotics to the body and harsh chemicals to the environment. Antibiotics play havoc with our body's natural immune system and are to be avoided whenever possible. Gargling with hydrogen peroxide kills cold and flu germs and whitens teeth.

· To clean pans of scorched rice or other carbohydrate foods, soak overnight in a solution of water and distilled vinegar.

- Another option to clean cooking pans is to make a paste of 1/4 cup baking soda, squirt with hydrogen peroxide and apply with fingers or a sponge.

- Distilled vinegar wiped on feet and the liners of shoes helps prevent and alleviate athlete's foot. Apple cider vinegar is an effective anti-fungal solution as well.

- Comfrey in a poultice was the healing method my husband Phil used after I experienced a burn on my arm from a treatment given me at the hospital. Phil made a paste of powdered comfrey root with a little honey and warm water. He spread it between two pieces of plastic wrap to roll it out. He peeled off one piece and placed the poultice against my arm burn. By morning the redness was subsiding and the area was beginning to heal. Phil used it to heal his broken rib, since there's little to be done with a broken rib but to give it time to heal itself. Phil's poultice of comfrey worked quickly.

Natural Toothpaste for a Clean, Healthy Mouth
==

Ingredients to combine:

3 Tbsp baking soda

1 Tbsp neem powder

3 Tbsp extra virgin coconut oil

1 Tbsp xylitol (for taste)

15 drops of mint essential oil (for aroma & breath)

Combine and prepare a paste. Store in a glass jar. Coconut oil may harden depending on the room temperature. This paste not only cleans and whitens teeth, it heals cavities.

CHAPTER FIFTEEN

Conclusion

MENTAL AND SPIRITUAL HEALTH

P HIL SPENT A GREAT DEAL OF TIME collecting information to share with his students about eating healthy foods. He was fond of sharing the following inspiration with his students:

THE GOLDEN RULES OF HEALTH

1. Stop putting poisons into the body

2. It takes 5–7 times the normal amount of nutrition to build and repair than it does to maintain.

3. Nothing heals in the human body in less than 3 months; add one month for every year that you have been sick.

4. Have moderation in all things.

5. Make peace with nature.

6. Live closer to God.

7. You must take responsibility for yourself and your health.

8. Eat as much raw food as possible.

9. Exercise regularly the rest of your life.

10. Practice and learn to understand completely Hering's law of cure which is *"All cure starts from within, out, and from the head down and in reverse order as the symptoms have appeared."*

It is said that cancer is a disease of the mind, body and spirit. A proactive and positive spirit will help the cancer warrior be a survivor. Anger, un-forgiveness and bitterness put the body into a stressful and acidic environment. Learn to have a loving and forgiving spirit. Learn to relax and enjoy life.

We must try to protect ourselves by learning how to manage and lower our stress levels, eat properly, exercise as. much as possible and practice our devotion to the highest good.

When we are attempting to retain or rebuild our health we must remember that it takes at least three months and even more to rebuild cells. Some people tend to change their diet and life style for a short time and think it isn't working so they go back to their old ways not giving the body the chance to rebuild.

We understand that cells can become damaged in numerous ways including through the use of alcohol, which is a poison; smoking; consuming junk foods, breathing smog; drinking toxic water; eating foods from contaminated soil; too much sun bathing; using tanning beds; experiencing radiation from electromagnetic sources such as televisions, old CRT computer monitors, microwaves and especially cell phones.

I feel concern for this generation. Our dear son, a Vietnam veteran, whom I spoke of earlier, died from prostate cancer. Though he did a lot of alternative things and improved so much that, thinking he was much better, began to slide back into his old eating pattern. Perhaps just as damaging to his body, he would sit with his laptop computer in his lap to continue his work.

I kept trying to explain to him that this was not good. Sure enough, the prostate cancer came back with a vengeance. Heartbreakingly, I can't help but believe his laptop use had something to do with it.

Not exercising regularly and not drinking enough purified water daily to stay hydrated can also destroy healthy cells.

Besides diet we must learn how to cope with life to avoid stress. I always admired my husband, he left his work in his office, making a list of what had to be done, the crucial things that had to be taken care of the next day and came home to relax. He had a very stressful job, developing rocket engines and it could have affected his home life also but he did not allow this to happen.

Depression and anger can have a detrimental effect on our hearts so we should take charge of our own lives and decide how we are going to cope with problems that we all seem to have to deal with. We can think positively or think negatively about any situation, it is our choice.

Exercise is so important. So many come home from the office or place of work, plop down, eat a dinner of carbohydrates and fat and turn on the TV until it is time to go to bed. Our bodies were made to move—to burn up the calorie intake instead of letting it accumulate in fatty deposits.

Heart disease, stroke and cancer are illnesses that can result in not taking care of our bodies. It is recommended that we can help to save our lives if we have early warnings. A body scan, done by certified technologists and evaluated by your medical doctor can save your life when detected early. By knowing what the problem is one can do research on how to overcome it. So much information is available to those who care about their health enough to do something about it.

It is noted that one out of two people have some form of heart disease. We can find out if we are at risk with a Cardio Pulse Wave Analysis. Apparently when your heart beats, it radiates a pulse wave down the lining of your arteries and this pulse wave travels to your fingers and toes and then back. The frequency and strength of this wave measures the overall health of your cardiovascular system.

We are told by Caldwell B. Esselstyn, M.D. that we can cure heart problems. Every year, more than half a million Americans die of coronary artery disease (CAD). Three times that number suffer heart attacks. In total, half of American men and one-third of women will have some form of heart disease during their lifetime.

Esselstyn explains that heart disease develops in the endothelium, the lining of the arteries. We read that these endothelial cells manufacture a compound called nitric oxide that accomplishes four tasks crucial for healthy circulation. It keeps the blood smoothly flowing, rather than becoming sticky and clotted and allows the arteries to widen when the heart needs more blood, such as when you run up a flight of stairs. Nitric oxide stops muscle cells in arteries from growing into plaque, which is the fatty gunk that blocks blood vessels. It also decreases inflammation in the plaque. The process that can trigger cholesterol build up.

Too much fat in the diet damages the endothelium cells that produce nitric oxide so it is recommended to have a plant-based diet as much as possible. I would add to this that live foods are so important because cooking destroys enzymes which are needed to digest our food.

I made the choice eight years ago when my cardiologist wanted to put me on Plavix and I refused. He informed me that I could die any time from a stroke or heart attack because I was a walking time bomb. I told him I was in my 80s and if I died it was time. I didn't want to put that in my body. I proceeded to change my diet and started a regiment of Omega 3, a product from Melaleuca Wellness Co., liquid Quinol CoQ10 from Costco, Cardiac plus, Orchex and Cataplex E from Standard Process Labs, digestive enzyme, Heart Plus and Superfood from Dr. Schulze's American Botanical and cayenne capsules from the health-food store. It is quite expensive but not compared to some of the medications that were prescribed. After insurance, I still would have to pay about $225 per month for one of the prescriptions.

I am still here, and my cardiologist tells me I am doing well now. Originally, my heart was enlarged, shaped funny and worn out, as he said and now the recent C-scan shows my heart is not enlarged nor misshapen. Perhaps this wouldn't work for everyone. We are all different but it worked for me. Even to change your diet even a little and think about what you put in your mouth will be for your good.

We are told that a plant-based diet may offer protection against stroke, high blood pressure, osteoporosis, diabetes, senile mental impairment, erectile dysfunction, and cancers of the prostate, colon, rectum, uterus and ovaries. If you value your health, it is worth a try to change your diet to feel better.

Jack Challem, of the American Society for Nutrition suggests we should avoid synthetic foods, they are manufactured not grown. Read labels. If you don't recognize most of what is on the label don't buy it. Find food grown without chemicals and GMOs. Genetically engineered seeds tolerate high applications of herbicides, specifically glyphosate, a possible carcinogen, which through chemical studies has been found in the urine of children and adults.

Work done by a Dr. Otto Heinrich Warburg, who in 1931 was awarded the Nobel Prize in Physiology/Medicine, looked at the relationship between acidic body chemistry, toxicity (caused by fermenting sugars) low oxygen and corresponding sub-optimal performance of the body.

In reading an October 2016 article by Sarah Cooke entitled "Nine Ways to Say No to Sugar", she stressed how detrimental sugar is to our health and that it is addictive. She suggests ways of possibly overcoming the sugar habit—by eating regularly so our blood sugar doesn't drop, and eating a little bit every few hours to prevent this from happening. Never skip breakfast—our blood sugar level is lowest in the morning. Never eat the sugar coated cereals. Usually fruit as it is easy to digest. I enjoy an apple and organic cheese. Eat whole foods, not processed foods that are loaded with high fructose corn syrup and many unseen sugars. Do not use the artificial sweeteners such as Spenda, NutraSweet, etc. Perhaps a little stevia or raw honey if fruit does not taste sweet enough. I sometimes add a little chopped pineapple or banana in my shredded wheat cereal with sunflower or almond milk, that I make myself, and it tastes sweet. One can use cinnamon, cardamom or cloves to help make food or drinks seem sweeter. Sarah Cooke mentioned in her article that we sometimes don't have enough "sweetness" in our lives, so we turn to sweets. We should try to engage in activities we enjoy. And if I may add, all work and no play is not healthy for us.

She states that we should love ourselves. Cutting out sweets feels like a sacrifice. We don't want to feel deprived. It is amazing to me that when I had cancer and lived on live foods—only having melon and granny smith apples, even the thought of chocolate cake or anything with sugar in it make me feel sick. I do eat some sweet things now, but nothing made with white sugar or corn syrup, etc. I use honey or maple syrup. I find it so easy to say no when everyone else is eating the bad things, I just think and feel badly because they don't know what they are doing to harm their bodies. I buy coconut milk ice cream and have a little occasionally, or I will bake a pie with a whole wheat flour crust, and sweeten the apples with a little raw sugar or honey and stevia. I never craved sugar and sweets as I did before when I eliminated all sweets from my diet. If I ever do eat something that is made with white sugar, I wake up at night with leg cramps and I think...*what did I eat?*

According to Dr. Linus Pauling, two-time Nobel Prize winner, "You can trace every sickness, every disease, and every ailment to a mineral deficiency." Minerals are the foundation to sound nutrition and health. We are told that mineral deficiencies are more common now as we mentioned before because of depleted soils and highly refined diets.

Phil loved to share the following anonymous poem with his students. It's a fitting way to close the book he so wanted to share with them as a takeaway reference source for having a healthy, happy life. He passionately believed every line of it.

What to Count

Count your blessings instead of your crosses;

Count your gains instead of your losses.

Count your joys instead of your woes;

Count your friends instead of your foes.

Count your smiles instead of your tears:

Count your courage instead of your fears.

Count your full years instead of your lean;

Count your kind deeds instead of your mean.

Count your health instead of your wealth;

Count on God instead of yourself.

—Author unknown

LIFE-CHANGING FOOD FOR OPTIMUM HEALTH

We Can't Live Without Water and We'll Live Longer and Healthier When We Consume Enough of It

SEVENTY-FIVE PERCENT of Americans are chronically dehydrated and it probably applies to half the world population. The thirst mechanism is so weak in 37 percent of us that it is mistaken for hunger. Even mild dehydration slows metabolism down 3 percent.

One glass of water will shut down nighttime hunger pangs for almost 100 percent of the dieters studied in a University of Washington research study.

Lack of water is the number one trigger of daytime fatigue. A mere 2 percent drop in body water can trigger fuzzy short-term memory, trouble with basic math, and difficulty focusing on computer screens or printed pages.

Drinking 5 glasses of water daily decreases the

risk of colon cancer, bladder cancer and breast cancer. Those risk decrease factors range from 45 percent to 79 percent.

How to Make Sole Water

The antibacterial and anti-fungal properties of the Sole will help make it last indefinitely.

- Fill a quart-size mason jar 1/3 full with unrefined natural salt.
- Add filtered water to the jar, leaving two inches empty at the top.
- Cover the solution with a plastic (not metal) storage cap.
- Shake and allow the solution to rest for 24 hours.
- Check in 24 hours to see if all salt crystals are dissolved and add a little more salt. When salt no longer dissolves, the Sole is ready.
- Store covered on a counter or in a cupboard.

How to Take Sole Water

- Add 1/2 tsp of Sole to an 8-ounce glass of filtered water (the water can be warm) each morning, before breakfast.
- Taste the Sole—if it tastes salty (like you would expect it to), then it is the perfect

amount for you.

· If it tastes too salty, dilute with plain, filtered water until it tastes just right. If it does not taste salty enough, add some more Sole until the balance is right. You have to trust your senses on this one—your body knows best!

The amount you need may vary each day.

When shopping for sea salt, look for an unrefined sea salt. Which retains all the natural minerals your body needs. Look for pink Himalayan salt or Celtic gray sea salt. Colima sea salt is great—but is not sold in stores.

Drinking a mixture of natural salt and water is nothing new. It has been used as a remedy around the globe for centuries. Table salt, of course, can be harmful. Most of the original natural minerals are removed with heat treatment, bleaching, and packaging. Compounds are added, such as synthetic iodine, anti-caking agents, fluorides, etc. All of these procedures and additives can cause significant health problems, such as elevations in blood pressure. So we are advised to limit our salt intake.

. . . . .

ALOE'S HEALING PROPERTIES

. . . . .

Aloe vera juice and pulp may ease digestive distress and decreased chronic inflammation. Breaking off a leaf and squeezing the gel directly onto sunburned skin is not only a healing moisturizer but its natural amino acids and salicylic acids reduce inflammation and "take the fire" out of a burn.

. . . . .

CAPSICUM OR CAYENNE RED PEPPER'S HEALING PROPERTIES

. . . . .

Cayenne is a medicinal and nutritional herb. The therapeutic action of cayenne is well documented: stimulant, tonic, astringent, antispasmodic, emetic, antiseptic, anti-arthritic, and others, and of course—condiment.

Cayenne cannot be equaled in stimulant strength by any known agent. It is effective in alleviating congestive chills, heart failure, diarrhea, dysentery and offensive breath. It heals ulcers, rebuilds tissue in the stomach, and helps digestion when taken with meals.

Cayenne pepper induces programmed cell death, a property lacking in cancer cells, meaning cells do not extend their life span and perish at the appropriate time. Unlike chemotherapy, **cayenne only affects cancer cells and the normal cells remain unharmed**. The capsaicin substance is known to arrest tobacco-induced tumors and is used to treat lung cancer.

Cayenne is an anti-fungal, anti-inflammatory and anti-bacterial substance. It is used with honey and lemon juice to detoxify the body. It is effective in treating tooth and gum diseases and is used topically to treat snake bites and other wounds. It also prevents blood clots, so is not advised for post-surgical patients because it may cause excessive bleeding.

· · · · ·

Top Whole Foods

· · · · ·

- **Almonds**—source of monounsaturated fatty acids, they boost good cholesterol while lowering the dangerous kind.
- **Avocados**—rich source of potassium and heart-healthy fats, a hunger fighter.
- **Blueberries**—rich in cholesterol-reducing antioxidants, anti-diabetic agent, enhanced memory and heart healthy.

- **Flax seed**—one spoonful provides 8 grams of omega-3 fatty acids, and packed with vitamins.

- **Kale**—source of vitamin A, promoting immune and eye health and cancer-fighting antioxidants.

- **Lemons**—A single lemon has more than 100 percent of a person's daily vitamin C requirement. Flavonoids act as anti-inflammatories and inhibit growth of cancer cells.

- **Pomegranate**—The seeds in one fruit contain 1.5 grams of protein. Pomegranates fight free radicals that contribute to cancer and other chronic diseases.

- **Quinoa**—This gluten-free seed contains more iron, fiber, protein and calcium than rice, oats or wheat.

- **Spinach**—One cup contains a person's daily requirement of vitamins A and K, and nearly 100 percent of manganese and folate.

- **Wild salmon**—source of omega-3 fatty acids to boost brain function, an abundant source of vitamin B-12, for red blood cell production and nerve function.

. . . . .

Foods That May Trigger Arthritis

. . . . .

wheat
dairy foods
corn
citrus fruits
tomatoes
eggs
sugar

. . . . .

Proper Food Combining

. . . . .

1. Liquids alone, or liquids first, then wait 1/2 hour to eat.

2. Do not combine dense proteins with dense starches.

3. Do not combine acid fruits with sweet fruits.

4. Fruits alone.

5. Melons alone.

- DENSE PROTEINS: nuts, seeds, avocado, coconut, meat, fish, and dairy.

- DENSE STARCHES: potatoes, grains, beans, peas, winter squash, artichokes, and corn.

- ACID FRUITS: citrus, plums, pineapple, strawberries, oranges.

- SWEET FRUITS: bananas, figs, dried fruit, prunes, persimmons.

- Eat as much of your food raw as possible. 80 percent raw and 20 percent cooked.

. . . . .

EVELYN FONS' TIPS FOR THE COOK

. . . . .

- Always leave the head or the root end on an onion when grating it to prevent cut fingers or knuckles or broken fingernails.

- Flax seed and water can replace eggs in quick breads, pancakes and muffins. Use 1/4 cup flax seed and 3/4 cup water, blend well and it will replace 3 eggs.

- Flour bacon before frying. The grease doesn't spatter and the bacon doesn't shrink as much. It has more body and a beautiful crust.

- To grease a baking pan, hold it upside down under hot water for a few seconds. The warm pan or dish can be greased easily and evenly.

- Stem and core apples carefully. Ninety-nine percent of the pesticides are in the skin.

- Walnuts are good for the brain, heart and

our bodies. It is not recommended for high-temperature cooking. Store walnut oil in a cool, dark place for up to 3 months. It is even best to keep it in the fridge to prevent it going rancid. (It's an excellent skin-softening solution too).

- Ketchup cleans copper tarnish from cooking pots and tea kettles.

- Add 1 tsp of pure apple cider vinegar to fruit or vegetable gelatin salads to keep them from running after being unmolded.

- Never soak fruits or vegetables in water for more than a few minutes so as to preserve vitamins and minerals.

- Drop frozen vegetables into boiling water while frozen; vitamin C is lost if they thaw before cooking.

- Mold spores in the refrigerator produce aflatoxins that settle on other foods. Keep all food covered. Wipe shelves and walls with damp paper towels after a misting of alcohol or a paste of water and baking soda on a weekly regimen.

- Wash strawberries in vinegar water to prevent mold, drain, and store in zip-lock plastic bags with a paper towel in each to absorb excess moisture.

· Use stainless steel for top of stove cooking and pyro-ceramic dishes for oven baking and roasting. I do not use aluminum because it leaches into food. I do not use Teflon, because at high temperatures it releases a deadly gas.

. . . . .

HEAT-SHOCKING PRODUCE PRESERVES FRESHNESS

. . . . .

Food scientists have discovered an effective way to extend the life and nutritional qualities of fresh produce.

Warm water—not scalding—but ranging in temperature from 105–140° F, to give fruits and vegetables a brief plunge, will firm their flesh, delay browning and fading, slow wilting and increase mold resistance.

This is according to W. Wait Gibbs, reporting for the *Associated Press*.

Washing pollutants and pesticides from fruits and vegetables, particularly strawberries, peppers and greens can prevent a lot of health problems.

A friend does this for fresh flowers before refrigerating them in her vegetable crisper drawer. The procedure makes them last a few days until she can arrange them for a dinner party.

· · · · ·

SPROUTING PRODUCES LIVE ENZYMES TO ENHANCE SALADS, SOUPS, SNACKS AND BREADS

· · · · ·

Mentioned in earlier chapters, sprouting seeds, beans and grains provides nutrients the body can utilize optimally.

- **Green peas**—protein, carbohydrates, fiber, vitamin A, iron, potassium, magnesium and chlorophyll.

- **Lentils**—protein, iron, vitamin C. Use in breads and salads.

- **Garbanzo beans**—carbohydrates, fiber, calcium, protein, magnesium, potassium, and vitamins A and C.

- **Black-eyed peas**—protein, vitamins A and C, magnesium and potassium.

- **Almonds**—protein, calcium, potassium, phosphorus, magnesium, organic fats, vitamins B and E.

- **Pumpkin seeds**—vitamin E, phosphorus, iron and zinc (essential and rare to find in our modern diet).

- **Kamut**—protein, magnesium, lipids, 16 amino acids, zinc, vitamin E and energy carbohydrates.

NOTE: *Do not use garden seeds that have been poisoned to kill insects. Purchase seeds from the health-food store.*

There are several methods of sprout growing. I like the wide-mouth quart jar with a screen top lid or use a nylon stocking with a rubber band over each jar.

How to Sprout:

Soak chosen seeds overnight in a large jar. (Some seeds such as sunflowers and sesame seeds don't need to soak that long, perhaps 4–6 hours is sufficient). To sprout, put 1/2 cup seeds or beans in a quart jar as above. Drain and lay the jar on its side with the lid covering as described above. Cover the jar with a towel to keep the contents dark. Rinse and drain several times each day.

When sprouts are obviously growing well, remove the towel and expose the jar to sunlight, so the sprouts will turn green to enhance chlorophyll production. I do this for alfalfa sprouts. It takes about 5 days before alfalfa sprouts, for example, are ready to eat. Rinse them with cool water and store in the refrigerator to stop growth. Rinse them occasionally while refrigerated to keep them fresh. Use quickly for their maximum nutritional value.

The following chart provides approximate amounts of various seed types, sprouting times, and yields.

SEED TYPE	AMOUNT	HRS TO SOAK	DAYS TO SPROUT	YIELD
Small (*alfalfa*)	1 Tbsp	overnight	5–7	2 c
Medium (*wheat*)	1/2 c	10–12	2–3	1-1/2 c
(*sunflower, radish, broccoli*)			4–6	
Large (*kidney*)	1 c	10–12	5–6	4 c

Seeds are the core of life. They contain generative power for growth. Sprouts are living food offering abundant nutrients, minerals, vitamins, simple sugars, amino acids and enzymes in easily digestible form. Best intestinal cleansers are alfalfa, fenugreek, lentil and mung.

Sprouts are inexpensive, always fresh and have the potential to help solve hunger and malnutrition problems in our communities and in developing countries. Sprouts are precious in winter when the quality of fresh fruits and vegetables is not is often compromised. Winter fruits and vegetables also are more expensive than when abundant fresh ones are in season.

I wish all parents could feed their children sprouts. They would save money and save on doctor bills, because their children would be healthier. Nursing mothers would do well to eat alfalfa and wheat sprouts, and drink sprout tea for extra nutrition. Adding sprouts to their and their children's sandwiches provides protein, iron and vitamin C. Add them to meat loaves, breads, salads and smoothies, too.

Sprout milk is nutritious too. Begin with one cup of wheat, sprouted for 2 days. Combine with 4–6 cups of purified water; blend for 2 minutes on high speed. Strain in a fine wire-mesh strainer. Discard pulp. Return liquid to blender and add 1/2 cup raisins. Blend and strain as before. Serve.

. . . . .

HONEYBEE POLLEN, AND HONEY THE PERFECT FOOD

. . . . .

Honey is the only food on the planet that will not spoil or rot. However, it will crystallize if left in a cool dark place for a long time. If this happens, loosen the lid, boil some water, and place the honey container in the hot water. Turn off the heat and let it liquefy. It will be as good as it ever was.

Honey is loaded with enzymes essential to our bodies. Our grandparents ate comb and all. If you can locate local honey that has not been commercially processed you will certainly be blessed with good health. Use it to sweeten foods and beverages and to heal. A mixture of honey and cinnamon cures most diseases according to some experts.

. . . . .

THE GREEN TEA SOLUTION

. . . . .

The heart is susceptible to threats from all around. Green tea has been proven to lower LDL cholesterol, lipids, and triglycerides—all contribute to clogged arteries and resulting in heart and circulatory problems. Green tea is an antioxidant.

Green tea helps protect bone-building cells from free- radical damage. It also fights the bacteria that cause gum disease. Green tea is also good for your brain, cutting back on the production of the protein called amyloid beta, implicated in Alzheimer's disease.

The National Cancer Institute published a study claiming regular green tea consumption reduced chances of developing esophageal cancer by up to 60 percent. It is touted as a weight-loss enhancer as well.

. . . . .

Rebuild Bones with a Smart Diet
and Exercise

. . . . .

Eat a diet rich in vitamin D and calcium to optimize bone building. As we age bone mass decreases. Sedentary lifestyles are destructive, favoring desorption of bone, creating muscle weakness, then a fall can be devastating. To avoid these problems, follow these suggestions:

- Dietary sources of vitamin D are: egg yolks, saltwater fish (fresh caught), liver and raw milk. Recommended intake is 400–600 IU daily.

- Dietary sources of calcium are: organic kale, dairy products such as raw milk, cheese, and yogurt; salmon, sardines, baked beans, sunflower seeds, and organic cereals.

- If you are lactose-intolerant, legumes will help.

- Strength training builds bone and fights osteoporosis.

. . . . .

Effective Nutrition Rebuilds Joints

. . . . .

Joints are made up of cartilage, bone and ligaments—all held together by the muscles surrounding those joints.

- **Cartilage**—cartilage serves as a cushion in your joints to prevent our bones from grinding together. It does not contain a blood or nerve supply so healing after an injury can be difficult. Vitamin C is good for cartilage growth, contributing to collagen production, the vital protein that makes cartilage. Citrus fruits, green bell peppers, strawberries, watermelon and broccoli are recommended.

- **Bones**—bones in our joints require us to eat calcium-rich foods.

- **Ligaments**—ligaments connect bones in our joints and are critical to our balance, movement and stability. Take quercetin, a bioflavonoid to ease inflammation. Onions are rich in quercetin. Eat foods high in vitamin C for collagen production. Zinc, oysters, crab, organic pork shoulder and cashews are rich in zinc.

- **Muscles**—healthy muscles are essential for rebuilding joints. Adequate protein is necessary for healthy, lean muscle.

A WEALTH OF HEALTHY RECIPES FOR TASTY FOODS YOU'RE SURE TO ENJOY

After you've won your cancer battle, consume 80 percent raw vegetables and fruits and 20 percent cooked foods. Add the following food items sparingly and enjoy! Phil and I have collected this array of recipes from a variety of sources. These are a few of our favorites.

Phil did not recommend using white flour—enriched or otherwise. He had a favorite saying that referenced the commercial companies taking out wheat nutrients and "enriching" the bleached flour with questionably sourced replacements:

"If I gave my wife a $20 bill and took it away and gave her a $5 bill instead, she wouldn't say she'd been enriched—she'd say she'd been robbed."—Phil Fons

White flour is not present in the following recipes, and it's not the only purposely-omitted ingredient.

Because soy is the most common genetically modified organism (GMO) in our food supply, we have omitted recipes calling for soy products as ingredients. Substitutes for common soy products include the following:

Soy sauce	Coconut or other. Aminos, beef, mushroom or vegetable broth, balsamic vinegar, fish sauce made with anchovies
Soybean oil	Avocado oil, olive oil, coconut oil, macadamia nut oil
Soy milk	Organic milk, almond, cashew, coconut, hazelnut or rice milk
Mayonnaise	Mayo made with avocado or olive oil
Edamame	Green peas, fava beans, chickpeas
Tofu	Mushrooms, chickpeas, cooked, cubed chicken pieces
Silken tofu	Vegan yogurt made from almond or coconut milk, sometimes combined with arrowroot powder as a thickener (as opposed to cornstarch, which is usually GMO).

. . . . .

TURMERIC PASTE HEALS

. . . . .

According to Dr. Arjan Khalsa, turmeric helps alleviate fibromyalgia, arthritis, muscle pain, parasites, bacterial infections and it aids digestion. It is effective in detoxifying the liver.

To make turmeric paste to use by the tablespoon in yogurt, juices, milk (cow or almond), rice, and salad dressing:

Basic Turmeric Paste :

1/2 cup purified water

1/2 cup turmeric powder

Mix water and turmeric in a small sauce pan on medium heat, stirring constantly until mixture is a thick paste. Cool, put in a small jar and keep in the refrigerator until ready to make milk.

Golden Turmeric Milk

2 cups coconut milk

1/2 tsp cinnamon

1 tsp coconut oil

1–2 tsp turmeric paste

1 tsp grated ginger

5 or 6 peppercorns

Pinch of stevia or honey, to sweeten

Simmer for 10 minutes, strain.

Serve with sprinkle of cinnamon; or to store: cool and add 1/4 tsp sesame, walnut or coconut oil and store in a glass jar.

Garlic the Healer

. . . . .

Known as *Allium sativa*, garlic fights off viruses and bacteria. Louis Pasteur noted in 1858 that bacteria doused with garlic died. It is a well-known infection fighter. The ancient Greeks advocated garlic for everything from curing infections, and lung and blood disorders to healing insect bites and even treating leprosy. It is true that garlic increases the overall antioxidant levels of the body.

All forms of garlic—raw or cooked—have the greatest biological activity of any single known food. Oxidation of a cut, crushed or cooked garlic clove leads to the formation of more than 200 compounds, 70 of which contain sulfur. Sulfur is garlic's active ingredient. It is a mineral constituent of insulin, cartilage, the anticoagulant heparin, and some B vitamins.

Try my recipe for Garlic Soup on page 186.

. . . . .

Walnut Oil for Food, Skin Care & Massage

. . . . .

Although walnut oil is used in cooking, it is expensive and has a low smoke point. For those reasons it is often not the preferred oil in the kitchen. It is, however, also an excellent skin-care oil that leaves skin soft, smooth and relatively wrinkle-free. Its major ingredients are the Omega-3 fatty acids easily absorbed by the skin. It is packed with enzymes specific to cleaning up the stomach and intestines as well. Because it goes rancid quickly, it should be kept refrigerated and used as soon as possible.

Walnut oil is free of synthetic chemicals. Its use in bath products, lip balms, lotions, massage oils and face and body creams is far preferable to the synthetic ingredients in most commercial preparations.

. . . . .

Further Readings

. . . . .

My husband compiled a list of books that tell how to prevent or overcome cancer and other illnesses. He suggested that before you submit to cancer treatments, you deserve more answers. Do research and find out what you are dealing with. You can get a second opinion just by listening and viewing a video by Dr. Lorraine Day, "Cancer Doesn't Scare Me Anymore". This video is available by calling 1 800-574-2437; from *Rockford Press,*

P.O. Box 8, Thousand Palms, CA 92276, or www.drday. com.

"*Diet For a New America*" is by John Robbins, who describes what mankind is doing to contaminate, pollute and toxify our air, water, soils and the foods we consume.

Studies of the impact of our environment on our bodies continue to be researched and reported.

Dr. Mercola and other wellness experts can also be found online and in the library to assist you with up-to-date information from continuous new research and health studies.

Stay current with new information as Phil C. Fons led by example—to be mindful and continue learning how to enjoy a life of optimum health.

<u>Garlic Soup</u>
Serves 4

26 garlic cloves, unpeeled (*for roasted garlic*)

26 garlic cloves, peeled (*additional*)

2 Tbsp olive oil

2 Tbsp (1/4 stick) organic butter (*grass-fed dairy-cow source*)

1/2 tsp cayenne powder

1/2 cup fresh ginger

2-1/4 cups sliced onions

1-1/2 Tbsp chopped fresh thyme

1/2 cup coconut milk

3-1/2 cups organic vegetable broth

4 lemon wedges

Preheat oven to 350° F. Place the 26 unpeeled garlic cloves in small glass baking dish. Add 2 Tbsp olive oil, sprinkle with sea salt and toss to coat. Cover baking dish tightly with foil and bake until garlic is golden brown and tender, about 45 minutes. When cool, squeeze garlic between fingertips to release cloves. Transfer baked cloves to small bowl.

Melt butter in heavy 2-quart saucepan over medium-high heat. Add onions, thyme, ginger and cayenne powder. Cook until onions are translucent, about 6 minutes. Add the roasted garlic, 26 peeled raw garlic cloves and cook 3 minutes.

— continued

(*Garlic Soup—continued*)

Add vegetable broth; cover and simmer until garlic is very tender, about 20 minutes. Working in batches, puree soup in blender until smooth. Return soup to saucepan; add coconut milk and bring to a simmer. Season with sea salt and pepper for flavor. Divide into four bowls.

Squeeze juice of 1 lemon wedge into each bowl and serve.

This soup can be prepared a day ahead. Cover and refrigerate. Rewarm over medium heat, stirring occasionally.

— — —

Lemon Garlic Humus

3/4 cup olive oil

3 Tbsp lemon juice

2 cups garbanzo beans (chick peas), rinsed and drained

2 tsp minced garlic

1/2 tsp fresh-ground clove

1/2 tsp salt to taste (garlic salt or Himalayan)

Combine ingredients in blender or food processor until smooth and spreadable consistency, chill until serving.

Cut into wedges pita bread or flour tortillas—seasoned with olive oil and spices. Bake at 350° F for 8—15 min., to desired crispness. Dip in humus.

— — —

Healing Root Vegetable Stew

> 2 Tbsp coconut oil, organic butter or ghee
>
> 2 large onions, peeled and diced
>
> 3 large red potatoes, scrubbed, diced into 1-inch cubes
>
> 3 large beets, scrubbed, cut into 1/4-inch pieces
>
> 2–3 stalks celery, chopped into 1-inch pieces
>
> 2–3 parsnips, scrubbed, chopped into 1/4-inch discs
>
> 3–4 carrots, scrubbed and chopped into 1/2-inch thick discs
>
> 2–3 turnips, scrubbed and sliced
>
> 1 Tbsp fresh, grated ginger
>
> 3 Tbsp fresh, chopped garlic
>
> 1 can organic black beans (*or beans of choice*)
>
> 1 can organic peeled, fire-roasted tomatoes
>
> 2–3 cups vegetable stock
>
> 1 bunch kale, washed, torn into bite-size pieces

In a large pot, combine ingredients, adding enough purified water to cover, if vegetable stock is not sufficient. Bring to a boil, reduce heat and simmer until beets, parsnips, carrots and turnips are tender.

Season with sea salt, cayenne, tamari or bottled organic enzymes and serve.

Note: Because salads and other raw and steamed vegetables are such an important part of our diet, we've added the following dressing recipe to enjoy when you want to renew your experience with salads, or with steamed fresh vegetables or sliced fresh fruits.

— — —

Almondy Pear Dressing

    1-1/2 cups pear juice

    2 Tbsp almond butter

    2 Tbsp chia seeds

Add juice and almond butter to blender and blend on high until smooth. Add chia seeds then blend slowly on low (just high enough to turn over) for 10 to 15 minutes. This turns into a delightful and creamy dressing that can be used over a salad or as a dip for upping your raw veggie intake!

— — —

Healthy Barley Drink
(good for lymph glands)

3 Tbsp barley in 1 qt water

Boil for 30 minutes, strain, to the liquid, add ground cloves and cinnamon to taste. Drink one quart per day.

— — —

No-Bake Healthy Sweet

1 cup peanut butter, 100% (no additives, sugars, or preservatives), creamy or crunchy

2/3 cup honey, raw

2 tsp vanilla, pure extract

2 cups oatmeal, quick-cooking

1/2 cup coconut, flakes,

1/3 cup unsweetened flax seed,

1/3 cup ground wheat germ

1/3 cup dark-chocolate chips

Combine ingredients, roll into balls or spread into flat glass dish, cut into squares to serve.

— — —

Chocolate Coconut No-bake Sweet Treat

    1 cup coconut oil (softened, if it's solid)

    1 cup 100% pure cocoa powder

    1/2 cup pure honey

Mix all ingredients well and spread into a plastic-wrap-lined dish and refrigerate until set. Cut into squares and serve while firm.

NOTE: *Do not allow these to sit at room temperature for long, or treat will be too soft to eat as a finger food.*

— — —

Whipping Cream

    1/4 cup organic dried milk, reconstituted with water

    1 tsp lemon juice

Beat to form stiff peaks. Cool several hours. Stir in honey and vanilla to desired sweetness and taste.

TIP: Add a little baking powder (the non-aluminum kind) to assure stiff peaks.

— — —

Trail-Mix Snack

    1 cup quick rolled oats

    1 cup shelled nuts of choice

    1/2 cup shredded organic coconut

    1/2 cup wheat germ

    2 Tbsp virgin olive oil, or coconut oil

    1/2 cup pure honey

    1/2 cup raisins

    1 cup dried fruit

Combine oats and dry ingredients. In a separate bowl, mix oil and honey. Stir in oat mixture. (Reserve fruit and raisins). Spread on baking sheet. Bake at 300° F until brown. Cool, break into pieces, and mix in fruit and raisins. Store in small batches in covered containers or easy-to-hike-with Ziploc® bags.

— — —

Do-it-yourself Gourmet Spice Blends

Thai Blend:

1/4 tsp garlic powder

1/2 tsp onion powder

1/2 tsp ground cumin

1 tsp ground coriander

1/4 tsp ground red pepper

1/2 tsp ground ginger

1/2 tsp ground cinnamon

Mexican Blend

1/2 tsp garlic powder

1/2 tsp onion powder

1 tsp ground cumin

1/2 tsp ground coriander

1/4 tsp ground red pepper

1/2 tsp chili powder

1/2 tsp cilantro

— — —

No-Cook Fudge

In food processor combine and pulse:

1/4 cup sesame seeds, raw

1 cup oatmeal, old-fashioned or quick cooking

1/3 cup dark-chocolate chips

1/4 cup honey

Combine ingredients, roll into balls or spread into flat glass dish sprayed with olive oil, cut into squares to serve.

— — —

Granola

2–1/2 cups oatmeal

1/2 cup sugar, raw

1/3 cup honey, raw

1/3 cup butter, from grass-fed cows

Mix well, spread on lightly-oiled cookie sheet. Bake 10 minutes at 325° F. Allow to cool, loosen and stir. Add raisins, dark-chocolate chips, chopped nuts of choice.

1/4 cup wheat germ

1 tsp vanilla, pure extract

Mix well. Serve crumbled over yogurt or with raw milk, or spray an 8-inch square pan with olive-oil spray; pat in mixture; refrigerate, and cut into squares to serve.

Carob Banana Milkshake

In blender, combine and spin until creamy:

4 cups almond milk

1/2 tsp pure honey, or molasses

1 banana, ripe

1/2 tsp peanut or cashew butter

3 Tbsp carob powder

add ice cubes for desired consistency

— — —

Carob Frosting

Cream together:

2 Tbsp butter or coconut oil

1/2 cup dried milk

1/2 cup carob powder

1/4 cup honey, pure

1 tsp vanilla, pure extract

4 tsp milk

Beat well. Add a drop of peppermint if desired.

— — —

Caramel Popcorn

    2 cups raw sugar

    I cup butter

    I/4 cup purified water combined with I/4 cup honey

    I tsp sea salt

Combine in a saucepan and boil for 6 minutes to form caramel. Remove from heat, stir in quickly—the mixture will foam:

    I tsp baking soda

    I tsp vanilla, pure extract

Pop 3 popper-fulls of your favorite popcorn kernels. I use a large stainless steel bowl to combine and stir in foamed mixture—or, spread popcorn on a baking sheet, pour caramel sauce over popped corn, and stir to coat. Bake 45 minutes in a 225° F oven, stir occasionally. Serve after cooling. (Form into balls if desired.)

— — —

Healthy Alternative Graham Crackers

3/4 cup unbleached organic all-purpose flour

1-1/2 cups whole-wheat graham flour *(Bob's Red Mill is the brand I use)*

1/2 cup raw sugar*, pulsed fine in a blender (*or substitute stevia)

1 tsp baking powder

1/2 tsp baking soda

1/2 tsp salt

1/4 tsp ground cinnamon

1/2 cup cold, organic unsalted butter, cut into small pieces (or cold coconut oil)

4 Tbsp raw honey

1/4 cup cold water

1 tsp pure vanilla or pure maple extract

Preheat oven to 350° F. In an electric mixer, mix dry ingredients together. Add the cold butter a few pieces at a time and mix until it resembles coarse crumbs or cornmeal. Add the honey, water, and vanilla (or maple). Mix until the dough comes together in a sticky ball.

Between sheets of waxed paper, roll the dough 1/2-inch thick. Chill for 1 hour, or until firm. Remove from paper. Lightly flour the dough and roll 1/8-inch thick. With a sharp knife, cut into 2-inch squares (or use cookie cutters to make shapes of your choice.

Arrange the crackers on a Silpat®, or parchment-lined baking sheet. With a fork, prick several holes in each cracker. Sprinkle with raw sugar crystals. Bake for 15 minutes, until lightly browned at the edges. Remove from the oven and let cool in the pan.

— — —

Honeyed Popcorn

In large bowl combine:

2 quarts popped corn

1 cup nuts of choice

1 cup raisins

In small saucepan, melt 1/4 cup butter over medium heat.

Add 1/2 cup honey and 1/2 tsp cinnamon. Cook until hot, stirring constantly to avoid mixture getting too brown.

Pour hot honey mixture over popcorn mixture, and fold to coat evenly. Bake in shallow pan at 245° F for about 45 minutes, until crisp. Cool slightly, serve.

— — —

Honey Marshmallows

    3/4 cup raw sugar, pulsed fine in a blender

    1 cup honey

    1/3 cup water

    1-1/2 Tbsp unflavored gelatin

    1/4 tsp salt

    1 tsp vanilla

    1/2 cup cornstarch (or arrowroot powder)

    1/2 cup raw powdered sugar

    2 cups walnuts or pecans (optional)

Put water in a small saucepan, sprinkle gelatin on top, let stand several minutes.

Place pan over medium heat and stir until dissolved. It is only necessary to melt the mixture—DO NOT BOIL.

Add honey, sugar, salt, and vanilla.

Beat with electric mixer until thick/tacky. It will turn marshmallow-white. Add nuts and fruit, etc. as desired.

Mix 1/2 cup each cornstarch (or arrowroot powder) and raw powdered sugar. Sprinkle mixture in the bottom of 7-inch square pan.

Do not refrigerate. Let stand a few hours at room temperature before cutting with a hot knife. Roll squares or shapes in powdered raw sugar or toasted, grated coconut or chopped nuts of your choice.

— — —

Zucchini Fries

Cut zucchini length-wise to desired thickness and length for fries. Brush evenly with olive oil.

In a plastic bag combine:

3/4 cups bread crumbs

1/2 cup or more parmesan cheese

1/2 tsp oregano

1/2 tsp basil

1/2 tsp thyme

1/2 tsp garlic powder

1/2 tsp salt

pinch of cayenne pepper

Add zucchini fries and shake to cover all pieces. Arrange on oiled cookie sheet. Bake at 350° F for 15 minutes; then broil 5 minutes (watch closely so they don't burn). Remove to a platter and serve.

— — —

<u>Fry Batter</u> (*for tempura, chicken or pork*)

- I cup organic flour (plus extra for dry-coating)
- I egg
- I-I/2 cup milk
- I/2 cup olive or coconut oil

Mix well. Coat vegetables/meat pieces in dry flour before dipping in batter, so the batter will stick better.

Deep-fry a few pieces at a time in your choice of oil. Check meat for doneness before removing from hot oil.*

Rest hot fried pieces briefly on paper towels before serving.

*NOTE: *I prefer olive or coconut oil, but you may also use peanut oil—these three oils have a higher smoking point.*

— — —

Roasted Sweet Potatoes

Makes 4-6 servings

    2 pounds sweet potatoes

Preheat oven to 425° F, then combine the following:

    1 tsp coarsely ground coriander

    1/2 tsp fennel seeds

    1/2 tsp dried oregano

    1/4 – 1/2 tsp dried hot pepper flakes

    1 tsp salt

Cut sweet potatoes into 1-inch pieces. Toss in olive oil to coat, then fold in the spice mixture.

Roast on center rack of oven for 20 minutes. Serve hot, with butter if desired.

— — —

<u>Peanut Butter Sauce</u> *(to serve over vegetables)*
Makes approximately 1-1/2 cups sauce

    1 cup water

    3 Tbsp pure peanut butter

    2 Tbsp lemon juice

    1 tsp hot pepper flakes (or more)

    1 Tbsp arrowroot powder (to thicken)

    1/4 tsp sea salt

    1/4 tsp sweetener *or* 1/2 tsp raw sugar (pulverized in a blender)

    dash of liquid aminos (either coconut or Braggs)

Combine in saucepan over medium low heat until smooth and thick. Drizzle hot Peanut Butter Sauce over steamed vegetables to serve.

— — —

Evelyn Woods Fons

EVELYN WOODS was born on October 30, 1926 and grew up on a farm in Emmett, Idaho. As a high-school student, she had a job as the school principal's secretary and worked evenings and weekends at a local grocery store. After graduation, she moved to Portland, Oregon and took a job as a secretary. She married and had one son, before divorcing and moving to Southern California in 1951. She attended business college and worked as an office manager for an advertising company for many years, doing the accounting for the agency as well, while supporting her son.

In her early twenties, Evelyn had polio, which affected her left leg. She took ballet lessons as therapy. Her ballet master asked her to be his partner in an act that he and his ex-wife had previously performed. Their agent booked engagements for them to perform at night, and she worked at the ad agency in the daytime.

Evelyn was 37 years old when she met Phil Fons. He was 41, and like her, he had been divorced. He kept asking her to marry him and she kept saying, "No." She was raising her son by herself and didn't want to "make another mistake". Phil kept insisting that, "If two people were ever right for each other, we are." She gave in and married him. Sometime during their marriage, he told her about this great act he had seen while attending a management dinner meeting. Evelyn explained a part of the act and Phil was surprised to learn the lovely dancer was his very own bride.

After 50-plus years of marriage, Evelyn often told Phil she was glad he was smarter than she was about them being right for each other. Their talents and abilities complemented each other. Phil appreciated Evelyn's talents and had a way of making her feel "so special".

Phil had been alone for many years and had always had to pay for his secretarial needs. After their marriage, he was pleased he had his own secretary—his Bride—as he called Evelyn. She typed all of his class notes and helped in research for his lectures. He taught his Dixie State classes for many years and at the age of 91 was losing his hearing. Evelyn attended his classes to help him, but kept telling him she was tired of being his ears. He retired and continued to develop the book his students were begging to have as a resource for their own health and well being.

The Fons couple had many happy years together, traveling extensively. They went on two cruises: Alaska and sailing to the Caribbean through the Panama Canal. Other world traveling took them to New Zealand, Rarotonga, Fiji, the Hawaiian Islands, Jerusalem, Jordan, Arabia, Yemen, Oman, South America, England and countries in Europe.

Phil had wanted to purchase a painting in Rothenburg, Germany. Evelyn told him to take a photo and she would paint it for him when they returned home. He took the picture and she kept her word. The painting still hangs in their living room. Evelyn has completed many commission paintings and has sold much of her work. Her painted mural of a Parisian street scene fills an entire wall in their living room. Tuscany, Italy sets the theme for their bedroom wall. Evelyn taught painting for Dixie College to the adult educational classes, and also taught in her home studio in Bloomington.

She has always loved to write, and wrote articles about her childhood life on the farm. Many of her articles and letters to the editor have been published in local newspapers. She read something that concerned her in the local *Green Sheet* in San Fernando Valley, California where she and her son lived. She wrote a response to it, which someone clipped and put on the bulletin board at Pierce College. Her son saw it and said, "Mom, all the kids are reading it!"

It is Evelyn's joy to have fulfilled Phil's dream of completing his book. Together, their labors toward this publication share his vast research and passion for healing humanity one person at a time—just as he was able to save the life of his Bride.

Phil Corrigan Fons

PHIL CORRIGAN FONS was born in Chicago on March 21, 1922. After his father's untimely death in a train/auto accident when Phil was 12, his mother raised him and his three brothers during the Depression. Phil graduated with honors from Morgan Park High School where he was a ROTC officer. He then attended Illinois Tech studying mechanical engineering. He was recruited by

Consolidated Aircraft of San Diego, where he received training in flight testing engineering of the B24 Bomber in 1941. He joined the Army Air Corp and worked in instrumentation until a health problem caused his medical discharge. He served as a Flight Research Engineer on the Ryan FR1 Fireball and the Navy Turbojet Engine and fighter plane, later the first Navy Turbo Prop airplane. He did research and development testing as a propulsion specialist of the first Turbojet engine afterburner, the Firebird, and the first aerial drone.

North American Aviation paid his UCLA tuition to complete a 4-year program in industrial relations, leadership and management development.

As a pioneer rocket scientist, he stood at the test console to make the first large liquid-propellant rocket-motor firing in the free world on January 28, 1950. He participated in research and development testing of the Redstone Engine that sent America's first astronaut, Alan Shepherd, into space.

Phil worked closely with German scientists Werner Von Braun and Walter Reidel, as well as spending several years as a senior research and development engineering supervisor working on the Apollo LEM Lunar Expulsion Module Engine. It carried Buzz Aldrin and Neil Armstrong to the first landing on the moon.

America recognized his contributions to the

aerospace industry with President Barack Obama's formal commendation, as pictured at right.

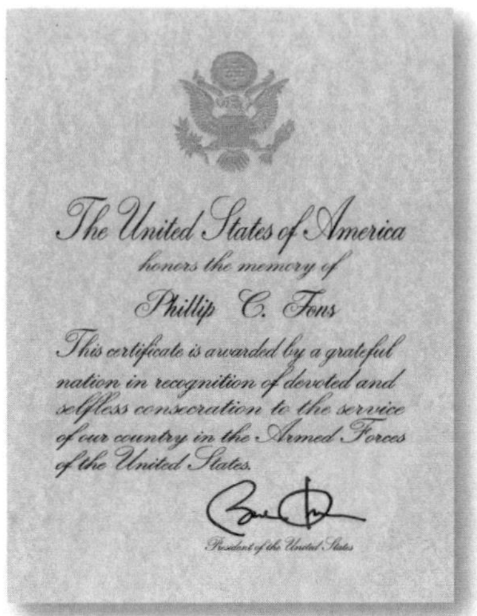

Phil was a respected scientific researcher at our nation's highest levels. It is not surprising a man with such a mind and so much determination and passion for good results should have succeeded in directing his wife's winning battle with cancer.

Now in his book, the rest of us can learn the life-sustaining ways we can prevent and cure disease by making informed choices for our own optimal health.